Caroline Hawkridge

CAROLINE HAWKRIDGE was diagnosed as having endometriosis at 23 and has remained well after having major surgery and 15 months of hormone treatment. She has been a trustee of the Endometriosis Society since its foundation, carrying out research, organising workshops and coordinating publicity. She currently works in health promotion for the Yorkshire Regional Health Authority, and has worked for the Health Education Council, the Open University and Leeds Polytechnic.

NICKY WESSON is a member of the Endometriosis Society and is the author of *Alternative Maternity* and *Home Birth*, both published by Optima in 1989. LESLEY MABBETT is a trustee of the Endometriosis Society and has wide experience of health education and community work.

DR STEPHEN KENNEDY, Research Fellow in the Nuffield Department of Obstetrics and Gynaecology at Oxford University, is currently involved in clinical trials for a new hormone therapy for endometriosis, and is developing new techniques for the diagnosis of the condition.

O P T I M A

UNDERSTANDING ENDOMETRIOSIS

Caroline Hawkridge

POSITIVE HEALTH GUIDE

© Caroline Hawkridge 1989

First published in 1989 by
Macdonald Optima, a division of
Macdonald & Co. (Publishers) Ltd

A member of Maxwell Pergamon Publishing Corporation plc

All rights reserved

No part of this publication may be reproduced,
stored in a retrieval system, or transmitted,
in any form or by any means without the prior
permission in writing of the publisher, nor be
otherwise circulated in any form of binding or
cover other than that in which it is published
and without a similar condition including this
condition being imposed on the subsequent
purchaser.

British Library Cataloguing in Publication Data

Hawkridge, Caroline
    Understanding endometriosis.
    1. Women. Endometriosis
    I. Title II. Series
    618.1'4

    ISBN 0-356-15447-5

Macdonald & Co. (Publishers) Ltd
66–73 Shoe Lane
London EC4P 4AB

Photoset in Times by 🅵 Tek Art Ltd

Printed and bound in Great Britain at
The University Press, Cambridge

Illustrations by Karen Huckvale.
Cover photograph by Raissa Page; Format 1.

CONTENTS

	Dedication and acknowledgements	vii
	Foreword	ix
1	Understanding your body	1
2	Understanding endometriosis	11
3	Drug treatments	35
4	Surgical treatments	49
5	Alternative and complementary approaches	65
6	Endometriosis and infertility	85
7	Endometriosis and pregnancy	99
8	Understanding your feelings	109
9	Getting to grips with pain	127
	Recommended reading	149
	Useful addresses	151
	Index	159

DEDICATION

For my mother, who had endometriosis before me, and my father, who convinced me I could write a book.

For Ailsa Irving, who had the courage to found the Endometriosis Society and changed our lives.

ACKNOWLEDGEMENTS

Recently I was asked what it was like writing this book. In some ways it was easy: I simply became a channel for women's experiences – fingers that translated their energy onto the page to be shared with others. I'd like to thank *everyone* who wrote with their stories. It just wouldn't have been the same without you.

Many people gave me support while I was writing. A very special thank you to Dr Stephen Kennedy and David Hawkridge who were entrusted with the red pen; your enthusiastic support and constructive advice were never ending! And to Ailsa Irving, Penny Broad, Diane Carlton, Lesley Mabbett and Kay Adcocks for further comments, Nicky Wesson and Lesley Mabbett for contributing Chapters 7, 8 and 9, Dr Anne Hawkridge for help with the anatomy and Dr Sean Hughes for raiding medical libraries. And a big hug for my old friend Karen Huckvale who did the illustrations; the menstrual cycle will never be quite the same again!

I'd like to thank the Endometriosis Society for making a survey of 800 members possible, Sharon Fordham and Roy Evans who spent so much time on the questionnaires and Indal Ltd. who generously gave us free computing facilities.

I am also grateful to friends who rescued me occasionally from the proverbial garret: Dr Brian Lake for our discussions, Francis Weir for poetry, Dave Newman and Stephen Cook for their life story and Jim Crook for being next door.

Last but not least, I owe a debt to my commissioning editor, Harriet Griffey, who supported my ideas immediately and has shared my excitement and panic ever since.

York, August 1988

FOREWORD

There is little worse in life than the misery of trying to endure intractable pain or prolonged infertility. Reading the pages that follow I sense that many endometriosis sufferers have had to endure such problems without much support. Life for many of them has become unbearable and their tragedy is compounded by the realization that no magical cure for their symptoms exists. Hence, they recognize the great need for self-help groups such as the Endometriosis Society which can provide relief simply by giving fellow sufferers an opportunity to share their experiences.

This book, compiled by members of the Society, is the first comprehensive attempt by sufferers in this country to convey their feelings, fears and anxieties about their symptoms and treatment. It tries to broaden the knowledge of doctors and endometriosis sufferers alike by giving a well-researched account of new methods of diagnosis and treatment. It differs from books written in the United States on the same subject mainly because women have different expectations of their respective medical systems which differ so radically. It is, therefore, more relevant to the British reader.

A recurrent theme throughout the book is the anger many women feel at the way they have been treated by the medical system and by society at large. I think this book will narrow the gap between some endometriosis sufferers and their doctors. It will demonstrate to sufferers some of the difficulties inherent in making an accurate diagnosis and in treating the condition. It will also serve to remind us as doctors just how debilitating a condition it can be. It is certainly an up-to-date account of modern research which, by branching out into disciplines such as immunology, is fundamentally altering many of our traditional notions about the cause of the condition and the causes of the infertility associated with it. The book also discusses the progress that has been made in the treatment of infertility through assisted conception techniques such as in-vitro fertilization (IVF). It will provide some much needed hope to couples who long for a child, by recounting stories of successful IVF treatments in women, for whom the idea of pregnancy seemed only a remote possibility.

The book explains medical facts in an easily understandable way; thankfully, however, it is deliberately not a medical textbook. It considers alternative forms of therapy, and the wider issues of being an endometriosis sufferer, in particular the adverse effects the condition has upon the psyche and upon relationships. More than anything else the book vividly describes what it feels like to have endometriosis: to cope with such emotions as the disappointment of failed therapy and recurrent disease; to suffer in silence the agony of painful periods and painful intercourse; to go through the stress of infertility investigations and treatment. Endometriosis is sufficiently common for these not to be rare events in our society. This is reason in itself for doctors to continue to research this condition which is still so poorly understood. There is much to learn: for example, we are only just beginning to appreciate that endometriosis may not be a disease confined to the pelvis but one that may have an effect upon the whole body. The next ten years will, I believe, see tremendous new developments in our understanding of the causes of endometriosis and in ways of diagnosing and treating it, all to the benefit, I hope, of sufferers.

Dr Stephen Kennedy

1

UNDERSTANDING YOUR BODY

Understanding endometriosis and its treatment is easier if you can imagine what you are like inside and how the menstrual cycle works. Understanding your body can be fun – and you don't need to be Einstein to get the basic idea!

HOW YOU ARE ARRANGED

Have you ever wondered how far apart your ovaries are? Or how big your uterus is? Or even what an ovary is like? Or how the menstrual cycle always happens in the right order over and over again?

A textbook chapter on the female menstrual cycle usually starts with a diagram in which the uterus is seen from the front

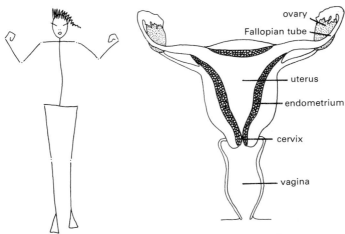

Getting to know your anatomy: front view.

with the fallopian tubes and ovaries stretched out on either side. Although this may be a convenient way to look at it in textbooks, it does not really help women to understand themselves. In reality the Fallopian tubes and ovaries are often tucked behind the uterus, which leans forward. The difference is much easier to imagine if you think of yourself standing upright with your arms outstretched, fists clenched into ovaries, as in the first diagram. To change to the position in the second diagram, bend forward at the waist and curve your arms behind your back near your sides.

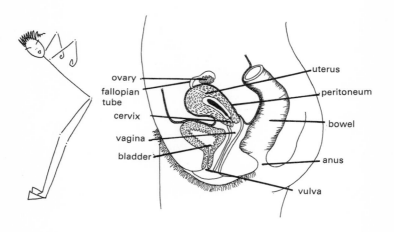

Getting to know your anatomy: side view.

Imagine yourself as a soft and floppy uterus from the waist up and that you are resting on the bladder which sits snugly in front of you while the bowel comes down behind you. The uterus tends to slide into different positions depending on how full the bladder and the bowel are. The uterus itself is about the size of your fist and each ovary is like a walnut.

If you imitate the uterus position shown in the second illustration you can feel your back muscles holding your body's weight as it leans forward. Similarly, your uterus also needs a means of support. The best way to understand this is to clench your pelvic floor muscles. If you are not sure how to do this, try the following next time you need to urinate. Sitting with your legs apart, stop the flow of urine in midstream and notice which muscles you use to do it. When you have got the feel of it, try it again later when you are not on the toilet – you can do it sitting down in the office or driving, standing up ironing or waiting at a bus stop. No one can tell! The muscles you are using are known as the levator ani muscles, although most people simply refer to them as the pelvic floor muscles.

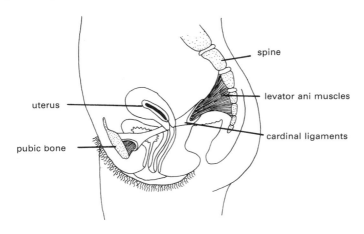

Levator ani muscles within cardinal ligaments supporting uterus.

The uterus is also supported by bands of elastic tissue known as the cardinal ligaments or transverse cervical ligaments. Some diagrams of the uterus often show the round ligament and broad ligament instead, although they are not very important. The round ligament is only a weak 'guy-rope' which is tightened to move the uterus forward. The broad ligament is not a ligament at all; it is a fold of peritoneum, the membrane lining the abdomen, and is easiest to imagine as a 'poncho' of fibrous tissue hanging over the uterus, with the ovaries like hands sticking out of the sleeves.

At this stage you might wonder why your uterus flops forward at all. It is not a stupid question. Think of the lower half of your body as a bucket, with the bottom taken out and replaced by a piece of canvas. The bones in your pelvic girdle are like the strong sides of the bucket and the canvas

Understanding the pelvic tilt.

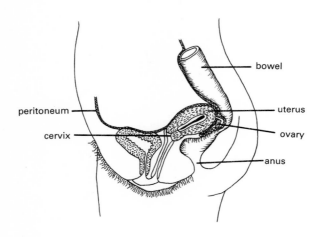

Retroverted uterus.

4

represents your pelvic floor muscles which stop you falling out of yourself! You would think the bladder, uterus and bowel would all be upright, and they probably would be if your pelvis was not tilted forward from your spine. As a result of this tilting, both the bladder and uterus flop forward under gravity, although the bowel tends to be held more upright as it continues up into the abdomen. You can get a feeling for your pelvic tilt by walking in high heels; this will force your pelvic girdle to tip forward more than usual, which in turn makes you walk differently.

Just to confuse the issue slightly, the uterus can be fixed in a 'retroverted' position. This is quite common amongst women in general, but is particularly common amongst endometriosis sufferers where the uterus has become stuck to the bowel with scar tissue (see Chapter 2). You can imagine the fallopian tubes and ovaries pushed up against the bowel in this position, although this is not always the case.

YOUR MENSTRUAL CYCLE

You are the expert on your own pattern of bodily changes during the menstrual cycle. You may have used charts to record your periods, your ovulation, and changes such as breast tenderness, irritability, bloatedness or differences in sexual feelings over the month. Most women would agree that these changes are to do with 'their hormones going up and down', but textbook diagrams which try to show this are usually rather daunting. The diagram on the next page combines a cartoon with some common medical charts to make them easier to understand. Do not worry if you cannot follow it all at first; the menstrual cycle is complicated and even doctors and scientists do not know exactly how it works.

The first thing to appreciate is that the pituitary gland (just below the brain) controls the menstrual cycle by sending messages to the ovaries. You are probably familiar with the idea of nerves carrying messages to and from the brain, but special chemicals also carry messages in the blood from one place to another. These chemicals are called hormones.

What happens in your menstrual cycle.

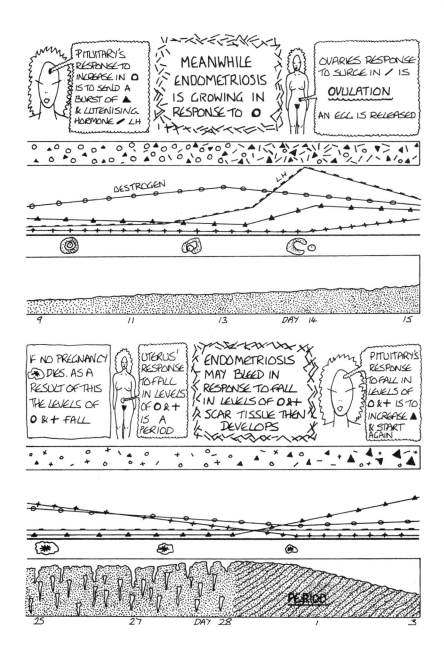

PITUITARY'S RESPONSE TO INCREASE IN O IS TO SEND A BURST OF ▲ & LUTENISING HORMONE ✓ LH

MEANWHILE ENDOMETRIOSIS IS GROWING IN RESPONSE TO O

OVARIES RESPONSE TO SURGE IN ✓ IS

OVULATION

AN EGG IS RELEASED

OESTROGEN

LH

9   11   13   DAY 14   15

IF NO PREGNANCY ✱ DIES. AS A RESULT OF THIS THE LEVELS OF O & ✝ FALL

UTERUS' RESPONSE TO FALL IN LEVELS OF O & ✝ IS A PERIOD

ENDOMETRIOSIS MAY BLEED IN RESPONSE TO FALL IN LEVELS OF O & ✝ SCAR TISSUE THEN DEVELOPS

PITUITARY'S RESPONSE TO FALL IN LEVELS OF O & ✝ IS TO INCREASE ▲ & START AGAIN

25   27   DAY 28   1   3

PERIOD

7

How hormones work

The way hormones work is easier to understand if you bear in mind a few simple ideas. Nerves tend to be like light switches; what happens will depend on whether they are on or off. Hormones are more like sounds since they can be on at different levels, so more varied and complicated messages can be sent. Organs such as the ovaries and the uterus are programmed to react in their own way to a change in the level of 'loudness' of a hormone circulating in the bloodstream.

Hormones and the menstrual cycle

The diagram on pages 6 and 7 illustrates how hormone levels change in a set pattern every menstrual cycle. Since the menstrual cycle repeats itself, you can start to look at what happens at any stage, but day 1 is usually counted as the first day of your period, with menstrual bleeding usually ending between days 4 and 7. Early in the cycle the pituitary gland releases more follicle stimulating hormone (FSH) into the bloodstream. One or other ovary will respond when FSH gets to a certain level. As its name suggests, this hormone stimulates a group of ovarian cells called a follicle to prepare an egg. At this stage the ovary starts to produce the hormone oestrogen.

Rising oestrogen levels mean different things to different organs. The uterus reacts by growing the lining (known as endometrium) to receive the egg, if it becomes fertilised. To the pituitary gland, the rise signals that an egg is being developed and that it is time to send a burst of luteinising hormone (LH) into the bloodstream.

The LH surge causes the follicle to release the egg (ovulation). Ovulation occurs around day 14, although this varies from woman to woman and may not be regular for the same person. It usually happens about two weeks before a period starts, so women with longer cycles also ovulate later. You can find out when you are ovulating by making a temperature chart. Ask at your local family planning clinic.

Once ovulation has taken place, the follicle turns yellow and is then known as the corpus luteum – translated as yellow body. The corpus luteum produces another hormone called progesterone, to make sure the endometrium – the lining of the uterus – is ready to receive the egg. Textbooks say progesterone makes the endometrium secretory; little sacks of

8

secretions develop which store food for the egg. If the egg is fertilised, it will plant itself into the endometrium and release its own hormone, human chorionic gonadotrophin (hCG), to make sure the body continues to look after it. Pregnancy tests are designed to detect small amounts of hCG that appear in your urine.

Unless there is a pregnancy, the corpus luteum only lives for a short time. As it regresses, the progesterone and oestrogen levels fall, signalling to the uterus to shed the endometrium, and you get a period. The pituitary gland reacts to the fall by increasing the level of FSH, and so a new cycle begins.

You may take the pattern of your menstrual cycle for granted, but it is very important from a biological point of view. The set pattern of hormonal messages between the pituitary gland and the ovaries ensures everything happens in the right order and at roughly the right time. For example, the egg will die if it arrives in the uterus before the lining – the endometrium – has been grown to support and nourish it. Your next period should only take place if you are not pregnant, otherwise you will lose the fertilised egg. Not surprisingly, the system can go wrong; ovulation or a period can be delayed by emotional upset, illness or poor diet, for example.

The way hormones control the menstrual cycle can be altered to prevent ovulation and pregnancy by taking the pill, which contains large doses of oestrogen and progesterone. When you stop taking the pill for seven days, the hormone levels fall and you have a 'period'. Doctors call this a withdrawal bleed because your body has been 'tricked' into shedding the endometrium by withdrawing the hormones. They often say it is not a real period because you would not have it unless you stopped taking the tablets. It may be lighter and less painful than your natural period.

Understanding your anatomy and the menstrual cycle will help explain where endometriosis is found and how it is affected by hormonal messages (see Chapter 2) and, in turn, how artificial hormones can be used to treat it (see Chapter 3).

2

UNDERSTANDING ENDOMETRIOSIS

He showed me on a model where the endometriosis was and that it was blood shedding itself. How it was getting there – behind the womb, just outside – I do not know.

The ectopic occurrence of endometrial tissue or its diffuse implantation or infiltration in the myometrium.
Stedman's Medical Dictionary

Even when doctors do have time to explain, endometriosis is not easy to understand. Women often feel confused but are reluctant to ask 'dumb' questions. And resorting to a medical dictionary is not usually much help.

This chapter explains what endometriosis is, how it is diagnosed and why there can be problems and delays. It also looks at who gets endometriosis and how it might be caused.

WHAT IS ENDOMETRIOSIS?

The word endometriosis comes from endometrium, the lining of the uterus. If you have endometriosis this means that patches of tissue a bit like the endometrium have been found growing in parts of the body where they do not belong. But rest assured, endometriosis is *not* cancer. It is usually found on the peritoneum – the membrane lining the abdominal cavity – and on the surfaces of the organs in the pelvis. The illustration on page 12 will remind you how the organs fit neatly side by side in the pelvis with their surfaces touching each other, more or less covered by the peritoneum.

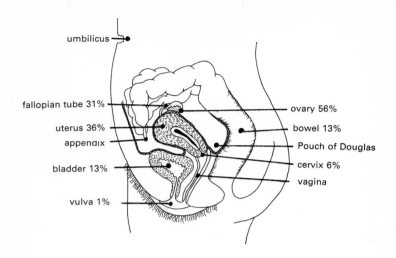

Where endometriosis can be found in the pelvis. (% figures from the Endometriosis Society Survey. Rarer sites — umbilicus and appendix — not in survey.)

Endometriosis often appears as clusters of bluish-black specks (rather like blood blisters). Patches on the ovaries are most common, but endometriosis can be scattered on the uterus and its ligaments, the Fallopian tubes, the bowel or in the pouch of Douglas. Other sites such as the intestines, appendix, bladder, behind the navel, on the lungs and on old surgical scars are far more rare. Occasionally endometriosis is found around the cervix, in the vagina or actually outside on the vaginal lips, and a few women have suffered from endometriosis in places such as the kidneys, pancreas or in more distant parts of the body like the arms, legs or head. In fact, a recent medical text notes an early record of endometriosis at Moorfields, the famous eye hospital.

If endometriosis is diagnosed in any of the above sites you will find it described in many gynaecology textbooks as 'external' endometriosis, because it occurs outside the uterus. 'Internal' endometriosis will be described as occurring inside the muscular wall of the uterus, and given the name adenomyosis. Researchers now no longer talk in these terms because they believe adenomyosis is a different problem — most women with adenomyosis do not have endometriosis anywhere else and it is much less common. Your medical dictionary may be equally out-of-date on this (see, for example, the dictionary definition at the beginning of this chapter).

Although patches of endometriosis are outside the uterus, they can still be reached by hormones in the bloodstream. Chapter 1 discussed the hormonal changes that occur during the menstrual cycle and the diagram on pages 6–7 illustrates how patches of endometriosis respond to these changes. Like normal endometrium, endometriosis grows in response to the female hormone oestrogen and may bleed slightly when hormone levels fall at the end of the cycle and your period starts (although this is not proven).

Inflammation often develops around these patches, causing pain. The peritoneum is particularly sensitive to this irritation. Scar tissue then forms around the patches, but each cycle involves more endometriosis growth and bleeding. Endometriosis on the ovaries can develop into 'chocolate' cysts – clumps of old blood which are either the result of monthly bleeding or an increase in blood vessels around the damaged site. These cysts have been known to reach the size of oranges.

Over time the constant build-up of scar tissue at different sites can lead to adhesions, best imagined as a kind of dense cling-film binding the organs together. Normally your organs slide gently against one another, but if you remember how neatly everything fits in the pelvis you can see how easily the ovaries might stick to the uterus or how the uterus might stick to the bowel, perhaps with one or both ovaries caught in between. Inflammation around endometriosis and subsequent adhesions can cause a range of problems.

SYMPTOMS

The symptoms emphasised in medical textbooks are one or more of the following:
- Infertility
- Painful periods (dysmenorrhoea)
- Painful sexual intercourse (dyspareunia)
- Painful bowel movements or urination

You might like to compare this with the table which illustrates what more than 700 sufferers said were symptoms of their

```
%        0  10  20  30  40  50  60  70  80  90  100
```

☆ PAINFUL PERIODS
    TOTAL MENTION — 94%
    MILD — 6%
    MODERATE — 22%
    SEVERE — 66%
    PAINFUL OVULATION — 77%
    SWOLLEN ABDOMEN — 77%
    LOSS OF STALE BROWN BLOOD — 72%
    PRE MENSTRUAL TENSION — 67%
    DEPRESSION — 63%
    LOSS OF LARGE CLOTS DURING PERIOD — 62%
    PAIN AT ANY TIME — 57%
☆ PAINFUL SEX — 59%
    HEAVY BLEEDING — 48%
☆ PAINFUL DEFAECATION — 48%
    CONSTIPATION — 45%
    NAUSEA — 42%
BACK PAIN
    DURING PERIODS — 37%
    MOST OF THE TIME — 42%
☆ INFERTILITY — 41%
    DIZZINESS — 33%
    IRREGULAR PERIODS — 31%
    DIARRHOEA — 29%
☆ PAINFUL URINATION — 26%
    INSOMNIA — 21%
    DUE TO PAIN — 32%
    PSYCHOLOGICAL SYMPTOMS — 15%
    OTHER — 13%

☆ TEXTBOOK SYMPTOMS

Symptoms described by over 700 sufferers in the Endometriosis Society Survey.

14

endometriosis in their opinion. It is striking how much pain many women suffer, whether it is severe painful periods (66 per cent), painful ovulation (77 per cent), painful sex (55 per cent), painful urination (26 per cent) or painful bowel movements (48 per cent). There is thus no doubt that endometriosis can in many cases be an extremely painful disease. Yet some sufferers do not have any symptoms at all. They may not even realise they have got endometriosis until it is discovered by accident when surgery is performed for a completely different reason – 8 per cent of women in the Endometriosis Society survey said their endometriosis was found during another operation.

Pain due to endometriosis probably relates to where the endometriosis is located rather than the amount involved. A large chocolate cyst on the ovary can be painless, while a small collection of growths in the cul-de-sac (Pouch of Douglas) may be responsible for very sharp deep pains during sexual intercourse – enough to spoil anyone's love life! Many symptoms of endometriosis are worse just before or during a period, when the disease may be more active. For example, you may notice that bowel movements or urination become painful at this time, and in severe cases blood may appear in your stools or urine. The regular build-up of inflammation and adhesions can lead to acute pain at any time or persistent pain throughout the cycle.

Pain is one of the most distressing aspects of the disease, capable of eroding your way of life, and affecting your confidence in yourself and others.

I *hate* the pain, it invades me.

I was convinced that the continued pain meant I would never recover and that I had not been told the truth.

On days free from pain or discomfort I feel great and can cope with any situation. When I do not feel well even answering the telephone is traumatic. I feel exhausted and my work is suffering.

Low energy level, lethargy and tiredness because of constant pain – day and night. Erratic mood changes. This general 'unreasonableness' was a major cause of conflict with my husband, also lack of interest in sex.

I know (in my case) my chances of pregnancy are small, but they would be much better if I could only get rid of the pain for a little while. I could then forget my non-pregnant state, relax more and give myself a better chance of conceiving.

It is clear from sufferers' comments that pain produces a lot of problems and these often combine to make them feel tired, miserable and out of control – 63 per cent in the survey said depression was a symptom of their endometriosis, 32 per cent complained of insomnia due to pain and 15 per cent mentioned various psychological problems. Most doctors would argue that tiredness and depression are not symptoms of endometriosis, but women count these feelings because they are describing what the whole experience of endometriosis can be like. For them, this includes problems caused directly by endometriosis, such as pain, and those it may cause indirectly, such as tiredness and depression. These feelings and ways in which pain and exhaustion can be managed are discussed in more detail in Chapters 8 and 9.

Another probable reason for the high level of depression reported in the survey is that 41 per cent had experienced infertility. Similar figures are given in other research. The association between endometriosis and infertility, and how women experience this problem, are explored in Chapter 6.

DIAGNOSIS

At present there is no quick simple test for endometriosis. Your doctor can check the position of the uterus and find certain signs that suggest endometriosis and exclude other possibilities during a pelvic examination.

Quite a lot of women have a retroverted uterus (see page 4) but this position is more common among endometriosis sufferers, where the uterus may be difficult to move because it is stuck to the bowel with adhesions. Your doctor may also be able to feel suspicious lumps, or that the ovaries are enlarged. Painful sexual intercourse is quite often associated with tender nodules in the cul-de-sac or uterosacral ligaments, so your doctor may try and reproduce this pain by prodding and stretching this area (be warned!). Sometimes thickenings in the ligaments due to patches of endometriosis can be felt if

Feeling the position of the uterus.

the vagina and rectum are both examined at the same time.

However, the best way to diagnose endometriosis is to see it. If you think back to where endometriosis is usually found (see page 12), you will realise that growths scattered around the pelvis cannot be seen by looking up the vagina – they can only be seen by looking inside the abdomen (except in rare cases where they occur beyond the pelvis). In the past this involved major abdominal surgery, but nowadays, a minor operation known as a laparoscopy is done instead.

Laparoscopy

A laparoscopy is usually a very quick operation under general anaesthetic, lasting 10–20 minutes. Carbon dioxide gas is pumped into the abdomen (they do let it out again) before an incision is made near the navel to insert the laparoscope, which lights up and magnifies the pelvic organs where endometriosis is usually found. Sometimes a second incision is made lower down and another instrument is used to move the organs slightly to look around and behind them. You will be in hospital for one or two days and may take a week or so to get back to normal after the operation. Your abdomen will feel tender and swollen at first, and there will be the usual after-effects of a general anaesthetic, e.g. possible nausea, tiredness, weakness. Some women complain of shoulder pains after a laparoscopy; this is because any carbon dioxide gas left behind will collect under the diaphragm (the sheet of muscle between the abdomen and the chest) and cause referred pain (pain felt in a different part of the body) in your shoulders.

Some assessment of the severity of the endometriosis will be made at laparoscopy. Medical texts outline ways of judging stages of endometriosis based on the number of sites and extent of adhesions. However this does not necessarily relate to symptoms; you may be diagnosed as having mild endometriosis, with a few patches in the pouch of Douglas or on the uterine ligaments, and yet be in agony.

Laparoscopy is now routinely performed to check the diagnosis of several gynaecological problems. The laparoscope is also used in infertility investigations and sterilisations. It is certainly a great improvement on major surgery of the past, but it is not an entirely foolproof method of diagnosing endometriosis. Endometriosis may be missed during the

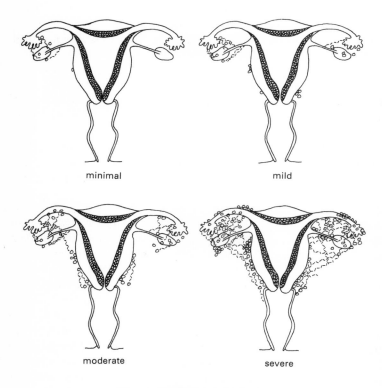

minimal   mild

moderate   severe

Degrees of endometriosis.

18

operation for various reasons. For a start, researchers have demonstrated that endometriosis can be microscopic – too small to see with a laparoscope. They are also beginning to agree that early disease may appear as colourless blisters, and the black colouration could be the end stage of the disease. And even if endometriosis is visible, it may be tucked away where it is difficult to see with the laparoscope, especially if adjacent organs are stuck together with adhesions. Adhesions in the absence of visible endometriosis could indicate other problems such as pelvic inflammatory disease (PID).

Some doctors have suggested that a laparoscopy for suspected endometriosis should be done just before a period, when the disease may be most active and easier to see. Although a few hospital wards try to ensure a woman is booked in late in her cycle, most do not make this special arrangement because of the lack of agreement on its value and the considerable organisation involved. Nobody knows how many women have not been diagnosed at their first laparoscopy because it was performed at an inappropriate time in their menstrual cycle.

A few gynaecologists are now advising a second look for women who have a negative laparoscopy (i.e. nothing was found) but who continue to suffer debilitating symptoms. One doctor reports finding the worst case of endometriosis he had ever seen at a second-look laparoscopy, when the first laparoscopy just nine months earlier showed a clear pelvis. This case is dramatic enough to prove the point, but in the absence of more information about how long endometriosis takes to become visible it is difficult for doctors to recommend when the second look should take place. Hospitals wishing to employ this strategy also have to cope with limited resources for re-laparoscopy and GPs' difficulty in making a second gynaecological diagnosis when laparoscopy has revealed nothing.

In some countries, particularly the United States, diagnosis is only confirmed if a biopsy (a small sample of tissue) shows endometriosis cells under the microscope. This procedure avoids mistaking other bleeding and blemishes seen during laparoscopy that are not due to endometriosis. However, a problem remains: Where do you take the biopsy from if you cannot see any endometriosis during laparoscopy? It is possible to take it from the wrong place and still miss the endometriosis.

Rare cases where women have endometriosis beyond the pelvis will also be missed at laparoscopy. These cases can be very difficult to diagnose unless *someone* notices the pattern of bleeding at these sites:

I had an ultrasound scan which revealed a large piece of tissue which was bleeding at the time (during my period). After a liver scan and X-ray which did not reveal a malignant lump, doctors decided that it could be endometriosis as it only seemed to bleed during my period causing severe pain and discomfort.

After coughing blood the chest X-ray showed a shadow on the lung – 10 days later it had disappeared. This continued for about 4 months and the chest physician was mystified as all other diagnoses had been ruled out. When I said to him how strange I thought it was that it occurred during the first few days of menstruation, bells started to ring and a gynaecologist was consulted. When the pattern had established itself over the next few months endometriosis was diagnosed.

An accurate diagnosis of endometriosis is important partly because treatment is different from that for other gynaecological or bowel problems with which it may be confused, but also because it is generally thought that endometriosis builds up inflammation and scar tissue every month if left untreated. A few studies suggest that endometriosis does not always get worse, but since doctors cannot predict who has progressive endometriosis and who has not, they cannot leave women to find out the hard way.

Future diagnostic tests

Researchers have been looking for ways to diagnose endometriosis without surgery, and one way is to look at the production of antigens and antibodies. The body's immune system reacts to 'foreign' chemicals (known as antigens) and invading infections by producing antibodies – chemicals of its own that clump around and try to neutralise or knock out the 'foreign' antigen or infection.

A blood test for endometriosis was suggested after high levels of an antigen, CA-125, were found circulating in the blood of some women with severe endometriosis. Further work showed that a CA-125 blood test could detect some severe cases, but other women had normal CA-125 blood levels in spite of having extensive endometriosis, and the test was even more unreliable in women with mild disease. Researchers are hoping to find another antigen produced by endometriotic tissue which will give a better test.

However, work in Oxford on CA-125 has been combined with a diagnostic technique called immunoscintigraphy. The idea is to give an injection of antibodies against CA-125 marked with a tiny, safe amount of radio-activity. The antibodies become concentrated in areas of endometriosis which can then be seen on pictures taken with a special machine that detects areas of radioactivity. This test does not depend on the levels of the CA-125 antigen circulating in the bloodstream, as the radioactive-labelled antibodies produced by the body go to the sites where the CA-125 is produced.

Researchers hope that immunoscintigraphy can be developed to detect endometriosis accurately, including disease that would be hidden or invisible (microscopic) at laparoscopy. Early work on ovarian endometriosis is promising, but it will be some years before the technique is fully developed and tested.

Getting a referral

Laparoscopy is not a simple test health centres can use to screen women, so it remains for your GP to arrive at a provisional diagnosis and refer you to a specialist for further investigation. To reach this stage both you and your GP have to agree that you have got a problem which needs specialist attention. You have got to respond to your symptoms by making initial or repeated visits; your GP must decide what your problem is likely to be and whether to treat you, refer you or ask you to come back if the problem persists. All sorts of delay can occur before you get a referral.

The Endometriosis Society survey tried to find out which symptoms prompted endometriosis sufferers to visit their GPs in the beginning. Replies suggest that infertility and severe period pains prompted sufferers to make the first visit more often than embarrassing symptoms such as painful sex or painful defaecation. For example, 66 per cent of women in the survey suffered from very painful periods and just under half

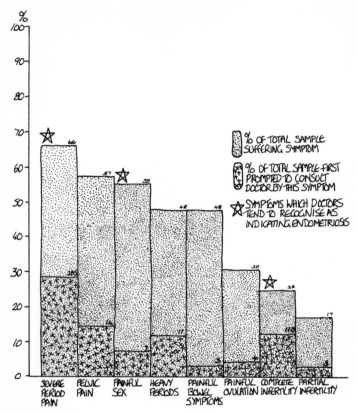

Legend

- % OF TOTAL SAMPLE SUFFERING SYMPTOM
- % OF TOTAL SAMPLE FIRST PROMPTED TO CONSULT DOCTOR BY THIS SYMPTOM
- ☆ SYMPTOMS WHICH DOCTORS TEND TO RECOGNISE AS INDICATING ENDOMETRIOSIS

RESULTS FROM ENDOMETRIOSIS SOCIETY SURVEY – 726 WOMEN

Symptoms first prompting women to visit their GP.

said this is what prompted them to visit their doctor. However 55 per cent suffered from painful sex, but only one in five of these women said this pain prompted them to seek medical advice.

Many sufferers also describe how they delayed going to their doctors because they thought their symptoms were a 'normal' part of being a woman:

> I just kept putting it down to other things, premenstrual tension, problems with relationships, the pressures of bringing up two young children.

22

Making love really hurt deep down in certain positions. I just thought, well, either he was too long or I was too short. How was I supposed to know? A friend said I ought to mention the pain to my doctor.

Some anticipated that their doctors would agree.

I feel doctors generally think pain is part of periods and we should put up with it – I thought this too, but it can mean that anyone with endometriosis does not seek help until it is really bad. What is bad pain? I always thought if I stand it then it must be bearable – maybe it would have been better if I'd fainted.

It can be very difficult to communicate your symptoms. Saying you cannot conceive is straightforward, but how do you convey just how much pain you are experiencing or how serious you feel things are.

My own doctor told me period pains were something women had to put up with, which infuriated me because I had explained that the pains I was having were far more than my ordinary period pains. I had not been able to conceive for two years and I was at the end of my tether with such dreadful pains.

You cannot produce proof of how you feel and therefore begin to wonder if you are exaggerating your symptoms when all the time you know you are being honest with yourself.

You may also be worried about your GP's response to 'feminine' complaints. The popular image of the neurotic female patient is all too familiar to endometriosis sufferers who feel their doctors did not take them seriously in the beginning. It is a recurring theme in stories of misdiagnosis:

Spastic colon, cystitis, neuroses.

Psychological – lack of commitment in my life!

Appendicitis, bowel spasms, chronic back pain, lack of sex causing congestion in the pelvis, retroverted uterus, over-active thyroid, neurosis.

He was convinced I had a kidney disorder. Everything else was in my mind. All he wanted to do was prescribe Valium.

Year 1: Stress, neurosis, psychosomatic.
Year 2: Menstrual troubles, 'will settle down', appendicitis?
Year 3: Ovarian cyst diagnosed by GP, consultant says I'm 100 per cent OK and tries to refer me to someone to 'talk about it'.
Year 4: Endometriosis.

'Suffering from acute depression' – that was what the doctor said. Seven hours later I was rushed into hospital and had an emergency operation in which they removed one ovary, one tube and appendix. Since then I found out they found endometriosis.

Many sufferers report that their doctors diagnosed their complaints as psychosomatic. The term 'psychosomatic' is often misused by doctors and the general public alike. Your doctor may mean there is nothing physically wrong with you and that it is all in your head (which is hysteria) or that you are exaggerating minor symptoms (hypochondriasis). Psychosomatic means your emotions (psyche) have produced a physiological effect on your body (soma). Psychological factors may contribute to the development of endometriosis (see Chapter 8), but this should not prevent recognition of a real physical disease requiring treatment. Equally, even if a woman is suffering from severe mental illness, she may still have endometriosis. Understanding is not helped by gynaecology textbooks which make statements such as 'girls' experience period pains because 'their outlook on sex, health and menstruation is faulty'.

Few women would deny that symptoms such as severe period pains or painful sexual activity are associated with emotional upset. However, they see this as the natural result of such pain, not the cause.

I felt a lack of knowledge and terror [about the pain] – which leads to neurosis which doctors then diagnose.

Several times over the last few years I have been told my problem is psychosomatic – a couple of years before endometriosis was diagnosed the doctor said the answer was to get married and have a baby! I felt so ill I burst into tears – which seemed to confirm the diagnosis!

One of the problems is obviously doctors' attitudes towards

women complaining of this sort of pain – they always seem to think 'She is neurotic, therefore she says she is in pain.' They never think 'She is anxious because she *is* in pain.'

The apparent contradiction between emotions and stress contributing to a disease on the one hand, and being a natural reaction to being ill on the other, is best understood as part of a vicious circle. For example, you probably will be anxious because you are in pain; equally your pain may also get worse as you become more anxious. These ideas are explored further in Chapters 8 and 9.

Even if you are able to communicate your symptoms and your GP keeps an open mind and is up to date, he or she may not refer you on your first visit. Endometriosis can be very hard to diagnose because individual symptoms vary so much and could indicate other gynaecological problems (such as pelvic inflammatory disease) or be mistaken for a range of bowel and bladder complaints (e.g. cystitis, spastic colon and irritable bowel syndrome). In addition, GPs are not experienced gynaecologists and do not have the benefit of a laparoscope, so short of referring every woman with painful periods to a specialist, many GPs wait and see if problems get worse and patients come back. This is illustrated in the Endometriosis Society survey, which showed that 41 per cent were only referred to a gynaecologist after repeated visits to their GP. Thirty-three per cent were referred straightaway, and this was more likely if the symptoms reported included infertility. The fact that 11 per cent were treated by their GPs for something else and 6 per cent were first referred to specialists other than gynaecologists may reflect lack of awareness of endometriosis, lack of up-to-date information and technical difficulty in making the diagnosis.

While 'wait and see' may be a reasonable strategy from your GP's point of view, it is tough on you if you are the one whose painful periods *are* due to a gynaecological problem such as endometriosis. You cannot do much about your GP's workload or medical education, but there are several things you can do if you feel you are not getting medical attention for the symptoms described earlier. The first thing is to go back to your GP; the survey shows that just because your GP did not refer you the first time, this does not mean he or she would not refer you next time. However this may be easier said than done when you have had to screw up your courage once already!

Fear and reluctance to discuss embarrassing symptoms are understandable but can also be counterproductive. In the absence of infertility, painful sex is one of the signs most likely to lead GPs to consider the possibility of endometriosis. Charting your menstrual cycle can provide useful information for you and your doctor since it will help you notice any changes. A pain scale (see Chapter 9) can help you record your pain. If possible, visit your GP when you actually have symptoms so he or she will be able to get a better idea of the problem. If you think you have got endometriosis, try suggesting it.

If you are concerned about your doctor's response then try writing down what you want to say. Plan to ask for what you feel you need (e.g. referral to a gynaecologist, pain relief, etc.). At least your GP may then give reasons if he or she does not agree, rather than simply not realising your concerns. Talk it over with a friend or partner beforehand to check you have thought it through. It may also help to take someone with you for moral support. If you have difficulty understanding what your GP says, ask him or her to repeat or clarify it. Make notes if it helps. If you do not think your GP has understood what you have said then check, or try repeating it a different way. If you do not agree with your GP's comments then do question them (yes, this can be hard). Doctors are human so being pleasant to them usually produces a better response (of course, this applies equally to patients!). Although it is easier to say nothing and perhaps accept tablets which you know you will not take, you will end up worrying and visiting your GP all over again. If you feel rushed into discussing things when you feel uncomfortable or embarrassed ('I would have liked doctors to talk to my face, not my bottom'), then ask for a minute until you are ready.

If all this seems impossible, then it may help to get some practice and support in being assertive. The most articulate woman who can stand up and talk to large audiences, run a playgroup or even take defective shoes back to a shop may come out of the surgery furious with herself for not saying what she meant to. Some people can only wind themselves up to say what they really want to if they get very angry or very upset, but they usually feel awful afterwards and this approach tends

YOU AND THE NHS

What you can expect as a right

- The services of a GP. You do not have to give reasons for changing doctors, but the new doctor is not obliged to take you. If no GP will take you on their list, apply to the family practitioner committee (FPC) who will arrange a GP to cover you for at least six months.
- To receive appropriate medical services, as judged by what other doctors would have done in the same situation, e.g. home visits.
- To be informed about substantial risks of treatment. Your consultant has wide discretion about what constitutes adequate information; ask about any treatment which is suggested.
- To have an abortion, sterilisation or any other operation without your husband's consent.

What you cannot expect as a right

- A home visit, if your doctor does not agree your circumstances require it in medical terms.
- A second opinion, although it is normally recognised as being an 'appropriate medical service'.
- To see your medical records, although you can expect them to be kept confidential from people not concerned with your treatment. You are entitled to see records held on a computer although they can be edited by your doctor first, and reports your doctor writes about you for employers, insurance companies, etc.

What you do not have to agree to

- Any particular medical examination or treatment. Treatment without your consent is assault, except in certain emergencies. Consent forms for operations are currently being improved. Discuss this with your doctor if you are worried.
- Having medical students present when you are examined. You have a right to be informed about this, and to be invited to give your consent. You also have the right to refuse examination under anaesthetic by medical students. These roles are under review.

to be counterproductive. Learning to be assertive can be extremely helpful and make you feel much more confident and positive (see the recommended list on page 149; assertive training courses may be available locally).

You may decide to change your GP. You can try seeing one of the other doctors in the practice or a locum – a doctor who takes over when your doctor's away. You do not need a letter from your GP to attend a family planning clinic, cervical cytology clinic or venereal ('special') clinic, so you could try talking to doctors there – they cannot usually refer you to a gynaecologist without your GP's consent, but a letter could carry some weight. If you do want to change your GP follow the directions on your medical card or ask your community health council (CHC) for help (address in the phone book). The local CHC is the patients' voice in your health district and is there to help you with problems and complaints. Ask them and other women about local doctors who may be more sympathetic to your problem.

WHO GETS ENDOMETRIOSIS?

Although most people have never heard of it, endometriosis is a common disease estimated to affect between 1–15 per cent of women. It is the second most common gynaecological disorder after fibroids, and is diagnosed in about 25 per cent of gynaecological operations.

Very few studies have looked at who gets endometriosis, if it is more common in certain groups, and whether there are risk factors which increase the chances of the disease developing. This kind of information could alert a doctor when making a diagnosis, and understanding risk factors can make prevention easier (e.g. recommending that women over 35 who are sexually active have a cervical smear). Equally, inaccurate information can hinder diagnosis and delay the decision to do a laparoscopy.

Endometriosis is associated with menstruation, so it does not occur before puberty. However, many doctors are not up-to-date with reports that endometriosis can occur in women after the menopause, whether it be natural or surgical, e.g. if a woman is on hormone replacement therapy (HRT) or if fragments of ovarian tissue remain after surgery. Although

28

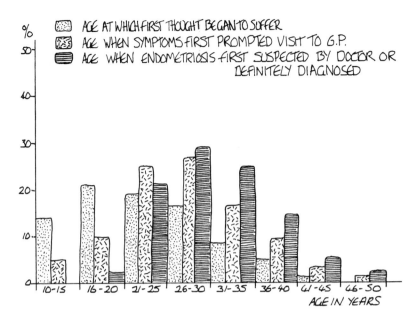

%
50
40
30
20
10
0

☷ AGE AT WHICH FIRST THOUGHT BEGAN TO SUFFER
▨ AGE WHEN SYMPTOMS FIRST PROMPTED VISIT TO G.P.
▤ AGE WHEN ENDOMETRIOSIS FIRST SUSPECTED BY DOCTOR OR
DEFINITELY DIAGNOSED

10-15   16-20   21-25   26-30   31-35   36-40   41-45   46-50

AGE IN YEARS

Age of sufferers when they felt they began to suffer, when they first visited their GP, and when they were finally diagnosed. (An Endometriosis Society Survey of 726 women.)

both these occurrences are very rare, women who had such an experience were not helped by their doctors' lack of awareness.

Endometriosis is often characterised as a disease most commonly suffered by white middle-class middle-aged women. This was quoted by the *British Medical Journal* as recently as 1980, in spite of the fact that supporting evidence is often drawn from clinical experience rather than research, and that studies have been published which contradict it. For example, work indicating that endometriosis is not rare in young women, including teenagers, has been available since the 1960s. There is more disagreement about endometriosis in different races; some studies suggest that twice as many white women are treated for endometriosis compared to black women and that it may be most common in oriental women.

He said I was far too young to have endometriosis [aged 22] as if somehow that meant I did not, even though he'd just diagnosed it at laparoscopy!

29

The hospital doctor did say that endometriosis was rare in Afro-Caribbean women.

Statements from clinical experience and research are limited to women who have been diagnosed. This is inevitable since you cannot find out whether endometriosis is more common in certain groups unless you know who has got it in the first place. But what about the women who have endometriosis and have not been diagnosed? Women with the disease can have no symptoms and be diagnosed by chance during an appendectomy or sterilisation. Endometriosis is difficult to diagnose anyway, and many sufferers report long delays in diagnosis. So perhaps endometriosis is more commonly *diagnosed* in certain groups. This explanation could account for some of the current statements about who gets endometriosis. For example, the suggestion that endometriosis is more common amongst higher social classes *could* be explained by the fact that these women often have the information and resources to get a diagnosis, perhaps by seeking private consultations more often.

The suggestion that endometriosis is a 'career woman's' disease, more likely to be suffered by women who have delayed child-bearing in favour of their job, is also controversial. There is no evidence that endometriosis is more common amongst career women and, since endometriosis is associated with infertility (see Chapter 6), a pattern of late pregnancies could be explained by reduced fertility amongst sufferers in general rather than choice of occupation. Continued use of the phrase is therefore unjustified and unhelpful, especially when it implies judgment on a minority of women who do decide to pursue a career in their 20s rather than have children.

Arguments about who gets endometriosis will continue for as long as it is impractical to screen all women for endometriosis. In the meantime, statements about the 'typical sufferer' are highly questionable.

Endometriosis in families

Research suggests that about 7 per cent of women with endometriosis have a close relative who also suffers. A similar proportion (8 per cent) of the 726 women in the Endometriosis Society survey reported endometriosis in their families. These figures do not necessarily mean that endometriosis is inherited; they might just mean it is so common that more than one person in a family will develop it. There is some research which argues that endometriosis is an inherited disease, although no one is sure why it only happens in some families and not others. And whenever it does, it can bring its own special problems and worries.

In June 1987 my younger unmarried sister started to complain of stabbing pains which were quite severe in her side. On hearing about me the consultant said she could have endometriosis. She went in for a laparoscopy and was found to have slight endometriosis. She has been put on danazol for 4–6 months. I have been able to help her, as no one was for me, by explaining things, reassuring, etc. My Mum is now blaming herself, which I keep telling her is silly. She is convinced that she did something wrong whilst she was bringing us up. I think she is the most upset of the three of us – one daughter having endometriosis was bad enough, but two!

When my endometriosis was discovered two years ago, my mother told me that she had suffered the same thing. She ended up having a hysterectomy where her consultant described the inside of her as if someone had taken a tube of glue and stuck everything together [adhesions]. I am the eldest of three girls but fortunately they have escaped it. I am hoping some research will be done on this as I have a beautiful young daughter (aged five) and would hate to think she will suffer in years to come.

One of the striking features of other stories is how much endometriosis can vary between sisters, or even between identical twins.

It is interesting to compare our symptoms – I had it very badly and no pain, my sister had lots of pain and only slightly.

I have an identical twin sister who has just been diagnosed, following painful periods for the last six months or so. I find it interesting that she has only recently developed the symptoms whereas my own endometriosis has been evident for nearly ten years now (we are both 29).

31

Of course, if members of families have similar symptoms, that can have disadvantages.

I finally screwed up courage to ask my mother about the deep sharp pains I felt during sex. She told me she'd had them for years and you could avoid them by only using certain positions. Later a medical friend said I should go and see a doctor. I told my Mom she should too. We both ended up having laparoscopies and endometriosis was diagnosed. I was 22, she was 47. So far my two younger sisters are fine.

WHAT CAUSES IT?

Medical theories

No one really knows why endometriosis occurs. There are plenty of theories which are difficult or impossible to test. The most popular one suggests the disease results from 'retrograde menstruation', when muscle spasms during a period force menstrual blood backwards up the Fallopian tubes and into the pelvic cavity, where it can form endometriosis. To understand how this can happen, it is important to realise that each Fallopian tube has a feathery end which opens out next to the ovary (see Chapter 1). There is a small gap between the ovary and the tube's entrance. Normally, when an egg is released it is guided across the gap and into the tube by the feathery 'fingers', and then passes on its way to the uterus. If menstrual blood is squeezed backwards up either Fallopian tube, it will leak into this gap between the 'fingers' and the ovary and then out around the organs.

The retrograde menstruation theory may explain why endometriosis is most commonly found on the ovaries, because this is the first place the stray menstrual blood is likely to land. However, research suggests that retrograde menstruation is common amongst all women, not just endometriosis sufferers. The theory does not explain why endometriosis occurs in the lungs and other distant places.

Another theory suggests that endometrial tissue is carried from the womb to other parts of the body via the lymph (fluid in the tissues) or blood, but again this does not account for why the condition only develops in certain women. Yet another idea, the metaplasia theory, states that cells in the body are converted to endometrial cells by recurring infection, hormone imbalance, or even outside chemicals.

Endometriosis has been reported in one or two men treated with female hormones for various cancers, e.g. cancer of the prostate gland. This observation tends to argue against the retrograde menstruation theory for obvious reasons and supports the metaplasia theory since cells must have changed into endometrial cells as a result of the high levels of the female hormones administered.

It has also been proposed that remnants of a woman's prenatal (before birth) tissue develop into endometriosis. At a very early stage in life, when a baby girl is growing in her mother's womb, certain cells are programmed to change into the female organs. It is thought that some of these cells can end up in the wrong place. When the girl begins to menstruate these areas respond to her hormones just like the normal endometrium because they came from the same foetal tissue.

There has been considerable interest in the more recent idea that women with endometriosis have an immune deficiency, i.e. the body's immune system is in some way defective. A weak immune system may allow endometriosis to develop as a result of retrograde menstruation or endometrial cells circulating in the lymphatic (tissue fluid) system, explaining why some women have the disease and not others. Some women with endometriosis have also been found to have unexpectedly high levels of antibodies which attack cells of some of their own organs, e.g. auto-antibodies to the thyroid. Immunology is a very complicated area of study so it will be some time before researchers can decide whether endometriosis is in fact an auto-immune disease and explain how it occurs.

Your theories

'Why me?' is a natural question when one is faced with a chronic, often painful, disease such as endometriosis. Most sufferers have some feeling about what caused their endometriosis, even if they just put it down to fate. In the Endometriosis Society survey, family history, stress (in general, a specific trauma or due to work), previous contraceptives, doctors' neglect, God's will and fate were most often ticked as possible influences on the development of endometriosis.

33

Women who replied to the survey were concerned about possible effects of the pill and IUD (the coil). There is no evidence that the pill stimulates the development of endometriosis; in fact some doctors have argued that it could have a protective effect, although this has not been confirmed by research. The pill may mask some symptoms of endometriosis by reducing period pains, but this has not been studied. The IUD often causes heavy, painful periods and some sufferers feel this led to their endometriosis. However many women get period problems with the IUD without developing endometriosis so, in the absence of research, it seems unlikely that the IUD causes endometriosis on its own. If you are worried about the pill or IUD then use another type of contraceptive for peace of mind.

Some women feel their endometriosis might have been caused by using tampons – a third of the 726 women replying to the survey said they had given up using tampons because of discomfort. It has been suggested that tampon use might increase the amount of retrograde menstruation and hence the chances of developing endometriosis. However, a study of tampon use amongst 470 members of the American Endometriosis Association found no evidence that tampon use was related to endometriosis.

3

DRUG TREATMENTS

My GP's comment was that I'll be better when I reach the menopause. With only 27 years to go, I can't wait!

There is no guaranteed cure for endometriosis, although it is rare for it to continue beyond the menopause. The fact that endometriosis does not grow and bleed if there is no menstruation means that drugs which stop menstruation can be used to treat it. Treatment usually lasts six to nine months and when your body returns to its normal cycle, endometriosis is less likely to recur.

This chapter looks at the drugs your gynaecologist may prescribe. Further surgery may be suggested in conjunction with drug therapy (see Chapter 4). What is recommended will depend on your age, your desire to have children (or more), where your endometriosis is and the problems it is causing. It will also depend on your consultant's views on endometriosis and its treatment, and his/her familiarity with new drugs undergoing trials.

DANAZOL

Danazol (marketed as Danol) was first described in 1971 and is now the most common drug treatment for endometriosis; 75 per cent of sufferers in the Endometriosis Society survey had taken it. Danazol tricks the body into a fake or 'pseudo-menopause', although it is uncertain exactly how the drug works. However the result is very low levels of the female sex hormone oestrogen.

If you are given danazol your periods will probably stop, although this depends on the dose, which may be anything from 200–800 mg per day. If your dose is too low you may get breakthrough bleeding as your body tries to have a period; most doctors believe that for the drug to be effective the dose should be high enough to stop menstruation completely (amenorrhoea). One or two women have reported taking doses as high as 1,200 mg per day; this is very high and if you are taking as much as this you should check with your doctor that it is really necessary. If you get any problems, discuss them with your doctor. There is no harm in you both adjusting the dose to find the right one for you – or in trying a different drug altogether.

You will usually be asked to start danazol after a period, to make sure that you are not pregnant – taking danazol during pregnancy can lead to a baby girl developing male characteristics. Danazol is only an effective contraceptive if taken at daily doses of 400 mg and above, so if you are taking less than 400 mg daily you should use a barrier contraceptive such as the condom or cap. Danazol is not recommended if you are epileptic, suffer from migraine, diabetes mellitus or heart, liver or kidney problems, and it should not be prescribed if you are breastfeeding.

Side effects

Danazol has a reputation for side effects and research suggests that 85 per cent of women are affected. Of the side effects reported in the Endometriosis Society survey, weight gain was the most common. Some side effects are related to the 'pseudo-menopause' danazol produces, e.g. hot flushes, dry vagina. Others, such as increased hair (hirsutism), acne and voice changes, occur because the drug is similar to the male hormone testosterone (but, you will be glad to hear, only one-tenth as strong). You will not necessarily get all these side effects or have them badly, and sometimes the number of side effects and their severity can be reduced by taking a lower dose.

Danazol arouses strong feelings amongst endometriosis sufferers. The side effects can be very depressing, but the relief from endometriosis or the subsequent pregnancy that results can make it all worthwhile. As with many other aspects of endometriosis, women tend to have different reactions and different needs. One has to balance side effects against relief of symptoms.

> I suffered shrinking breasts while taking it, but I still feel the benefits of being pain-free far outweigh the disadvantages.

> The side effects of danazol were tolerable. I am thin anyway, so I didn't mind the weight gain, although my face looked puffy. I also had hot flushes, but these were OK. I found remembering to take the tablets worse than the side effects.

Some sufferers have found that vitamin B6 and/or evening primrose oil (see Chapter 5) help counteract feelings of depression and lethargy when on danazol. Others comment that dolomite (magnesium/calcium) helps with muscle cramps.

> I would like to give some encouragement to people taking danazol. I have been taking 200 mg per day. I have offset feelings of depression and lethargy to a certain extent with vitamin B6 and have managed to keep my weight steady after an initial half-stone gain. I'm generally feeling better and more energetic and able to cope with life. The added bonus is no periods – even on this low dose. I have found that modifying my diet to eat more fruit/veg and natural yoghurts has also been beneficial – more fibre, fewer bowel problems and fewer spots.

Most side effects usually disappear when treatment ends, but it is generally accepted that singers should not take danazol because the voice changes that occasionally occur are not always reversible.

Not enough is known about other rare effects of danazol and their reversibility. For example, one sufferer reported problems with her contact lenses and then a drastic deterioration in her eyesight, which her optician associated with fluid retention in her eyeballs due to danazol. Fortunately, her sight returned to what it was previously when she abandoned the tablets. This case was dramatic enough to lead to use of the yellow card system, whereby the doctor notifies the possible side effect (of any drug) to the Committee on the Safety of Medicines. It may be more difficult to convince your doctor to report a severe side effect if it is chronic or a long-term aggravation of a previous complaint.

The Endometriosis Society followed up more than 300 women with persistent problems that might be related to danazol treatment. The vast majority complained of joint problems which developed while taking danazol, and in many cases the joint pain did not improve when they stopped taking it. It is not possible to conclude that danazol is responsible for this effect on the basis of an informal study, but until further research is done the findings do suggest it might be wise to choose another drug treatment if you already suffer from joint pains, or change to another drug if such problems develop.

Effectiveness

Whatever side effects you experience on danazol, you will want to balance them against its benefits. So how effective is danazol? It depends on how you judge success. For many sufferers it may be having a much longed-for baby. Reports of pregnancy rates after danazol treatment vary as the studies are not carried out in the same way; for example, different criteria are used for assessing how bad the endometriosis was, different treatment regimes are compared (e.g. sometimes surgery is performed as well) and different doses are given. To complicate findings, there may be additional reasons for a couple's infertility besides endometriosis (e.g. lack of ovulation, partner's low sperm count).

It is thus difficult to predict which women should have most hope of becoming pregnant. A 1985 summary of international studies reported that 31–53 per cent of those with mild endometriosis and 23–50 per cent of those with moderate endometriosis became pregnant after treatment with danazol. In general, women with mild endometriosis have a better chance of conceiving, but a few women with severe endometriosis have had some wonderful surprises.

I went in for a laparoscopy and they told me I might not be able to have children. I was very upset. The endometriosis was extensive. I had to take danazol for a year and then went back for another laparoscopy, which showed most endometriosis was gone. I was told I should try for a family. I had one period in June and then while on holiday in August realised I was pregnant! Our 10 lb son was born in April and I was over the moon. It was a difficult birth and they say the next one will be a caesarian, but I'm looking forward to it.

I was diagnosed as having widespread severe endometriosis after years of debilitating period pains. The endometriosis was found to be covering both ovaries, tubes, uterus, ligaments, bladder and in the cul-de-sac. After the laparoscopy my gynaecologist told me it was the worst case of endometriosis he'd ever seen and that if my husband and I wanted children we should put our names down for adoption. He suggested I take 600 mg per day of danazol for six months, followed by a laparoscopy to check my condition. During these months my husband and I came to terms with the fact that we would probably never have children and rearranged our lives accordingly. At the second laparoscopy, the gynaecologist found no evidence of active endometriosis. Just to make sure, I continued on the danazol for a further three months. To the delighted surprise of everyone concerned, I conceived just three weeks after ceasing the medication – a true miracle. My daughter is now a typical four-year-old with a delightful little sister. I had a few side effects while taking danazol – about half-stone weight gain, stomach upsets and deepening of my voice which is the only effect that has remained. If I found the endometriosis had recurred I would have no hesitation in taking danazol again.

The next big question is does danazol help the pain? There is a lot less research to answer this. It is easier for researchers to find out how many women were able to get pregnant after taking danazol rather than recording subjective measures of pain. One American review says that danazol relieves pain in 90 per cent of patients.

Out of all the treatments I received, danazol was found to be the most effective. It was highly successful as far as I was concerned and for the first time in years I was totally without pain.

Recurrence

The pros and cons of danazol would be easier to weigh up if it worked once and for all. But this is where the term 'recurrence rate' enters the debate because, as one medical author put it, 'patients need to clearly understand that hormone therapy of endometriosis will not result in a "cure" of the disease'.

The chance of symptoms returning after danazol treatment

varies from one woman to another. An often-quoted American study suggests that if symptoms do recur, this is more likely in the first year after treatment – 23 per cent recurrence, compared with 5 per cent and 9 per cent in the second and third years respectively. Another study indicates that recurrence may be higher amongst women who take a low dose (54 per cent recurrence in the first year after taking 100 mg/day).

A recurrence can be devastating, especially if pain was your main symptom.

Danazol for nine months. Pain completely gone. I could actually touch my toes for the first time in six years! Four months after stopping danazol, World War III broke out in my back! Returned to hospital for removal of left ovary. OK for another year. Gradually started feeling unwell – low backache, tiredness, heavy tender breasts, painful sex, trouble with bowels . . . danazol for eight months. Needed stronger dose (400 mg/day) to control and stop pain, which it did. Had problems with leg and muscle pains, so started taking water tablets [diuretics to reduce fluid retention] as well. Other side effects: weight gain, spotty, hair on head became very curly. Four months after stopping danazol, World War IV broke out in my back! Now control pain with alternative medicines.

Reading this story, one can understand how women end up taking danazol for far longer than initially planned. Little is known about the long-term effects of danazol, but even less is known about long-term use. Few cases are documented, yet some women contacting the Endometriosis Society have been on and off danazol for years in an effort to cope with their symptoms.

I started taking danazol 600 mg daily for nine months for severe endometriosis pain in my right groin, thigh, abdomen and back. I had very few side effects and it was effective immediately. Unfortunately, the pain occurred as soon as the danazol was discontinued and a total hysterectomy with removal of right tube and ovary was performed. To my horror the endometriosis pain was still present after the surgery. The gynaecologist who operated said 'it couldn't possibly be endometriosis now'! A second opinion confirmed that endometriosis was still present. Danazol was prescribed long-term because of my age – I was then 40 and the possibility of an early menopause (taking over as a natural cure) – and also because it would avoid further major surgery, for example, removal of remaining ovary and surgical menopause. I was prescribed 400 mg daily, reducing gradually to a maintenance dose of 100 mg which I am on at present. I feel fortunate that I have only experienced mild side effects – oily skin, decreased breast size, slightly deeper voice and mild hirsutism [increased body hair]. I realise there may be unknown, long-term side effects, but I feel that quality of life and not quantity is important. *If* danazol is going to cause problems later, then I must remember I have taken the drug by choice because it enabled me to live an active and enjoyable life which I was unable to do ten years ago.

This story illustrates the need for far better drug treatments of endometriosis. No one should have to carry the burden of long-term hormones with unknown effects. If you are taking danazol long-term, recent recommendations are that your doctor should regularly take blood to test your liver function and blood fats (lipids). The first test is important because danazol causes the liver to produce extra proteins. The second test is thought necessary because danazol *may* increase the risk of coronary heart disease, especially in women who smoke, are overweight, get little exercise or have a family history of heart attacks. Some doctors feel that non-androgenic progestogens (the progestogens are the group of sex hormones that include progesterone, and non-androgenic means they do not have male effects), such as Duphaston or Provera (see below), are a better choice for long-term use because they affect blood fats less.

Whether or not symptoms will recur after danazol is a hard question to face when you have spent six to nine months taking your tablets in good faith. No wonder doctors (and authors) wish they had more answers. There is only one way to find out, and if you have problems, whether it be after a few months or ten years, you will have to reconsider your options. Facing this uncertainty and the knowledge that endometriosis is a chronic (long-term) disease arouses deep feelings which you may need to share (see Chapter 8).

Side effects of drug treatment reported in the Endometriosis Society Survey.

The chart shows a scale from 0 to 100 %.

Side effects listed (top to bottom):

- WEIGHT GAIN
- TIREDNESS/LETHARGY
- BLOATEDNESS
- DEPRESSION
- NAUSEA
- HOT FLUSHES
- GREASY SKIN/HAIR
- HEADACHES
- DIZZY SPELLS
- DECREASE IN BREAST SIZE
- INCREASE IN BODY HAIR
- NIGHT SWEATS
- LOSS OF LIBIDO (SEX DRIVE)
- MUSCLE CRAMPS
- ACNE
- BREAKTHROUGH BLEEDING
- TENDER BREASTS
- ABDOMINAL CRAMPS
- SKIN RASHES
- HAIR LOSS

Legend:

DANAZOL — 545 WOMEN IN SAMPLE ALL DEFINITELY DIAGNOSED

PRIMOLUT N — 135 WOMEN IN SAMPLE ALL DEFINITELY DIAGNOSED

DUPHASTON — 126 WOMEN IN SAMPLE ALL DEFINITELY DIAGNOSED.

PROGESTOGENS

Primolut N and Duphaston

Primolut N (norethisterone) and Duphaston (dydrogesterone) are related to the female hormone progesterone. Technically they are known as progestogens, a general term for substances with effects like those of the natural hormone progesterone. Assuming you take a high enough dose, they stop your periods by tricking your body into a fake or 'pseudo-pregnancy'. These drugs are less commonly used (only 20 per cent in the Endometriosis Society survey had taken Primolut N and 20 per cent had taken Duphaston) but they may be a good second choice if you cannot get on with danazol. The side effects are generally less severe (see page 42), although progestogens are well-known for PMT-like side effects, e.g. bloating, irritability. Tender breasts are a particularly common problem on Duphaston. Breakthrough bleeding is also more of a problem than on danazol.

> After surgery I was put on danazol which had severe side effects, so my doctors suggested Duphaston instead. I kept getting breakthrough bleeding, even when I went up to the highest dose. I gave up and changed to Primolut N. Nine months' treatment finally did the trick and I have been free of symptoms for the past five years.

Provera

You may be surprised to be offered Provera (medroxyprogesterone acetate) if you have heard arguments surrounding the use of Depo-Provera as a long-term contraceptive in the Third World or the debate about the risk of cancer. Provera is the tablet form and does not have the same reputation for leading to a delay in fertility after its use as the injectable Depo-Provera. Some endometriosis sufferers have found Provera helpful, especially where other drugs have failed.

If you would like to try Provera but are concerned about it, then talk to your doctor and read around the subject before you make your decision (Write to the Women's Health Information Centre, page 152.)

THE CONTRACEPTIVE PILL

It may be suggested that you try taking the pill continuously (rather than stopping for a few days in between packets). Taking the combined pill (containing both oestrogen and progestogen) mimics pregnancy more closely than Primolut N or Duphaston because it prevents ovulation but with raised oestrogen levels. Doctors usually recommend a brand with a high level of progestogen (e.g. Eugynon 30) for endometriosis.

The pill's side effects are well known, but breakthrough bleeding is often a problem if you take them continuously. In many cases the dose is not enough to prevent spotting and women have found that severe symptoms of endometriosis remain. The pill can help keep mild symptoms at bay without the need for 'stronger' treatment, although the usual restrictions on long-term use in women over 35 and smokers still apply.

DRUGS IN CLINICAL TRIALS (IN 1988)

GnRH analogues

A gonadotrophin is a hormone that acts on the gonads (ovaries or men's testes). In women, gonadotrophin releasing hormone (GnRH) causes the release of two gonadotrophins, FSH and LH, from the pituitary gland, which in turn cause the menstrual cycle to progress (see Chapter 1). (GnRH is sometimes simply called LHRH – luteinising hormone releasing hormone.)

Recent research has produced a new family of synthetic hormones related to GnRH. Known as GnRH analogues because they have the same basic chemical structure as natural GnRH, these drugs interfere to such a degree with the release of FSH and LH from the pituitary gland (see Chapter 1) that they stop the menstrual cycle. This effect is known as a 'medical oophorectomy' because your body reacts as if the ovaries had been removed (oophorectomy) and it can be reversed by stopping treatment (i.e. 'medical' rather than surgical). So in other words you have a reversible fake menopause.

Clinical trials on GnRH analogues have been going on in several countries, including the UK, for some time now. New

44

members of this family of drugs keep appearing as different drug companies develop their own versions. Most of the research so far has been on buserelin, nafarelin and goserelin (Zoladex). Decapeptyl is less well known. They are usually taken by sniffing a spray or by placing a small implant under the skin.

GnRH analogues tend to have fewer side effects than danazol, although this varies from one woman to another. Women often experience some menopausal symptoms, e.g. hot flushes, dry vagina with consequent pain during inter-course, loss of libido (interest in sex), headaches and depression. All these symptoms disappear after treatment ends, including the small amount of bone loss that can occur (as it does after the menopause). Researchers are trying to prevent bone loss by adding progestogen to the treatment. Though they may have fewer side effects, GnRH analogues are not necessarily a more effective treatment for endomet-riosis than any other drug. Long-term studies looking at recurrence rates are not yet available.

I'm 31 and have suffered abdominal pains and discomfort from a very early age. Other symptoms were nausea, tiredness, depression and a permanent feeling of lethargy – symptoms were so bad they were ruining my social and working life. I went to see a consultant who diagnosed endometriosis. I was offered a chance to participate in the buserelin trials. The drug is in a nasal spray and very easy to use. I began to feel better almost immediately and my periods ceased after two months. Life became more meaningful and happy again. The only side effects were hot flushes and a few pains in my side. After six months a second laparoscopy revealed that nearly all traces of endometriosis had disappeared. It is now four months since treatment finished and unfortunately a few symptoms have returned, although thankfully they are not nearly so severe.

I'd suffered from endometriosis, painful periods, ovulation pain and pain at other times for five years. After nine months on dydrogesterone (Duphaston), endometriosis was no better. I had a laparoscopy and was put on goserelin (Zoladex), starting the third day of my period and given as a monthly injection of an implant just under the skin of the abdomen – a 'short sharp shock' which was soon over, sometimes leaving a small bruise. The first month I felt worse! Apparently the oestrogen level rises at first* so I had a painful cycle and a heavy period. Then the oestrogen level was suppressed and periods stopped completely – and hot flushes started. I had about 10–15 per day. I found it difficult to sleep at night. I had a slight weight gain of 4–5 lb but no other side effects. After six injections I was still having some pain. I had another laparoscopy and was told it showed no active endometriosis – very good news. The hot flushes stopped six weeks after the last implant and periods returned two weeks after that. Six months later I am feeling much better but still have period and ovulation pain. I'd say it was worth having goserelin (Zoladex). Although I am a little disappointed with the result, it was better for me than surgery or danazol which were put to me as alternatives.

Gestrinone
Gestrinone is another new drug undergoing trials. Its effects on the hormonal changes in the menstrual cycle are similar to danazol, but it only needs to be taken twice a week in 2.5–5 mg doses to prevent periods. At first glance this seems a dramatic improvement on taking tablets every day, but twice a week may be even more difficult to remember. Tablets are prescribed for six to nine months, but researchers are also hoping to produce gestrinone as an implant placed below the skin which would provide a year's treatment in one go.

In common with other new drug treatments for endometriosis, gestrinone offers a choice to women unable to tolerate danazol.

As danazol was not suitable for me, my gynaecologist agreed to me taking gestrinone for six months with regular monthly check-ups. I found it much more bearable, although there were some side effects – a skin irritation which was worse at night, some weight gain on my arms and legs which seemed to become more muscular. My breasts became smaller and my legs and face became hairy. After treatment, I had a laparoscopy which showed no evidence of endometriosis, but now three years later I am once again seeing a gynaecologist with suspected endometriosis. Although I

* Yes, this is, in fact, the case.

have suffered great pain, I am luckier than some women because I have two wonderful children, although at times they have been fed up with Mum not feeling well or being away in hospital.

So far, the information about side effects and recurrence rates is limited. Side effects are similar to danazol, although there are suggestions that not as many women suffer from them for as long or as badly. Most side effects are temporary and can be reduced by altering the dose or having an implant which is a better way of absorbing the drug (although your doctor has to put it in and replace it). However the one or two studies which look at recurrence rates are rather small and most statisticians would not take results from 20 patients too seriously.

4

SURGICAL TREATMENTS

Endometriosis can cause problems which do not respond well to drug treatment, so your doctor may suggest major surgery of one sort or another, e.g. laparotomy, hysterectomy. In the near future lasers and other instruments adapted for use down a laparoscope could make major surgery less necessary.

This chapter looks at what operations you may be offered, although, as with drug treatments, the advice you receive will depend on your particular case of endometriosis and your gynaecologist, who will not necessarily be familiar with the newer surgical techniques. This chapter also examines the issue of hormone replacement therapy after removal of the ovaries.

LAPAROTOMY

In general, drug treatments have little effect on ovarian cysts and large areas of endometriosis or adhesions (scar tissue), so you will probably need surgery to remove them. At present this is usually done during a laparotomy, a major operation to open the abdomen compared to the quick look with a laparoscope.

A laparotomy means a week to ten days in hospital, followed by at least a six-week recovery period. The incision is usually below the bikini line and becomes more or less invisible once it has faded. Any ovarian cysts (either blood-filled chocolate cysts or other fluid-filled cysts) and visible patches of endometriosis will be removed – unless, of course, this means removing an essential bit of you. Alternatively, the patches may be cauterised (heat-treated) in an effort to destroy them.

49

The surgeon will usually try and separate adhesions holding one or both ovaries in the wrong place. This can bring dramatic relief from painful intercourse if the ovary has been stuck down and bumped at all the wrong moments.

My doctor said I had a cyst the size of a hen's egg on my left ovary and recommended a laparotomy to remove it. They managed to free the ovary which was stuck down by adhesions between the uterus and bowel. I was amazed that my worst symptom, deep pain on intercourse, was gone! I was later put on danazol for remaining endometriosis.

You may have a ventro-suspension done at the same time, which involves tightening the round ligament although doctors disagree about whether this is worth doing since it is a feeble support at the best of times. Regular pelvic-floor exercises (see page 2) are probably far more effective.

There is no doubt that surgery is a good way to deal with large patches of endometriosis, remove cysts and separate adhesions in severe cases, but there are several reasons why surgery will never be a complete answer to endometriosis. For a start, the surgeon will only be able to remove or cauterise what he or she can see. There is mounting evidence that endometriosis is often microscopic, and the visible black 'powder burns' are only the end stage of the disease in a particular place. Even visible endometriosis can be difficult to recognise at times; for example, an ovary with a patch of endometriosis can look remarkably like an ovary bloodstained after a follicle has ruptured and released an egg.

Even if the surgeon is sure he or she can see the endometriosis, it may be in a very delicate area such as near the bowel or ureters (tubes which carry urine from each kidney to your bladder), where the risks and consequences of accidental damage are too great. Equally, the chances are slim of separating a uterus stuck against the bowel by extensive adhesions without causing worse damage. Doctors often recommend a course of hormone treatment after a laparotomy to make sure that any endometriosis that is hidden or impossible to remove gets a dose of treatment (and they may also suggest you take drugs before the operation to reduce the amount of endometriosis).

There is a debate about the value of surgery to separate adhesions and 'tidy the pelvis up', as the operation itself could cause more adhesions. Obviously, incisions result in scar tissue as part of the body's normal healing process, and the peritoneum which lines most of the pelvic cavity (see page 3) is very sensitive to all kinds of disturbance; for example, there is considerable evidence that old-fashioned methods of operating, which involve handling the internal organs with gloves dusted inside with talcum powder, lead to irritation of the peritoneum and build-up of adhesions. The aim of new microsurgical techniques is to use special instruments and particularly diligent procedures to minimise damage to surrounding tissue and, hence, later adhesions.

Microsurgery

Microsurgical techniques are becoming more popular amongst surgeons, although your gynaecologist may not have been introduced to them. Microsurgery requires special tools and meticulous procedures. For example, the organs are handled as gently as possible, using instruments rather than gloved hands. Metal instruments are Teflon-coated to give a non-stick surface to reduce abrasions, and smooth glass hooks are used instead of clamps and stay-sutures (stitches to keep things in place during the operation). Incisions are made using a microelectrical tool with a hot wire tip which seals as it cuts. Patches of endometriosis and small bleeding vessels are also sealed in this way. The area is constantly irrigated or washed with a special solution to rinse and cool treated tissues. Any debris is removed, along with the rinse, by suction. Care is taken to remove large pieces of tissue in one go rather than risk 'losing' bits which the body then has to clear up itself. Any stitching (e.g. to reshape the ovary after removing a cyst) is very precise and edges are folded in to make neat seams. Although these methods mean that the surgeon has to be very careful, methodical and even long-winded, they can have dramatic effects simply because the old adhesions have been separated and are not replaced with new ones.

If such care is not taken, the resulting problems with subsequent adhesions can be dramatic and debilitating. For example, Mary had a hysterectomy at 39, followed by removal of her ovaries a year later; though little endometriosis was evident at this time, extensive adhesions were noted by the surgeon. Endometriosis never bothered her again, but over the next few years problems with the accumulated adhesions really began.

51

The gastrointestinal pain gradually worsened. The diagnosis this time was duodenitis and hiatus hernia. Treatment did give a little relief but by January I was severely incapacitated and living on painkillers. At a laparoscopy no endometriosis was detected, but they found extensive adhesions on the bowel. My gynaecologist didn't want to operate as he felt major surgery would probably lead to even more adhesions within six months. He suggested that when I became bed-bound we would all have a rethink. I *was* virtually bed-bound and unable to perform normal housework; walking upstairs was a nightmare. Persuaded by my friends in the self-help group, my husband and I sought an appointment with a microsurgeon through my GP. By now my GP was confused and baffled, but felt an appointment couldn't do any harm. The surgeon allowed us to explain the problem and then described his procedures. My impatience to get on with it were matched by his understandable desire to check for himself that the gastrointestinal problems were negative. After two months he was convinced, and I was admitted. When I surfaced from the anaesthetic all the pulling pain had gone and the surgeon left me with a lovely smile saying he was quietly confident. Ten weeks later I was doing things I had not done for years without pain – walking, gardening, making love and, best of all, picking up my grandchildren! A slow but sure invasion of my body by adhesions – all alleviated by a few hours of tedious surgery. Life at 51 is wonderful!

HYSTERECTOMY

If you do not wish to have children (or any more) and you are in your 30s or 40s, then your gynaecologist may recommend a hysterectomy, although women in their 20s with very severe cases of endometriosis have also been offered hysterectomies.

Hysterectomy means that your uterus and cervix will be removed. Your doctor may suggest your ovaries are removed (bilateral oophorectomy) at the same time, but this is a much bigger step than a hysterectomy. You may also hear terms such as total hysterectomy, vaginal hysterectomy, etc. Many books and several hospital leaflets give more detail about the type of operation (as well as post-operative exercises and how to recover – see Recommended Reading on page 149), but do check with your doctor if you are not sure what is being recommended. Ask him or her to draw a diagram so that you know exactly what is planned.

The usual practice during a hysterectomy is to preserve the ovaries, but as one text puts it 'the question of whether to perform oophorectomy at the time of definitive surgery for endometriosis is difficult to answer'. If you are left with your ovaries (or one ovary, or even part of an ovary) after the operation, they will go on producing hormones, including oestrogen. If you have not reached the menopause, these hormones will ensure you continue with your menstrual cycles, so you may still feel PMT or familiar changes in breast tenderness, although obviously you won't have periods any more and you won't be able to get pregnant (even though you will be ovulating). The catch is that as long as you carry on producing oestrogen there is a chance that it will stimulate any remaining endometriosis. Patches may have been left behind, either because they weren't visible or they were on an important bit of you.

One review states that 'preservation of a normal ovary is associated with a 5–10 per cent chance of post-operative recurrence'. If this is generally true, between five and ten sufferers in every 100 having a normal hysterectomy will find that endometriosis returns in time. Turning this statistic on its head, it also means that the vast majority do not have any further problems, but you should be made aware of the risk before the operation to help you make your decision and avoid any nasty surprises.

> Why was I left to work out the diagnosis for myself when symptoms returned almost two years later? I thought I'd gone mad as I'd had my hysterectomy and here I was with terrible 'period' pains.

It is even worse if you get a bad recurrence and your GP can't believe it either because he or she is not up to date.

> One GP said my paralysing cyclical pain two years after hysterectomy (earlier appendectomy) was due to 'colic' and greeted it with heavy sarcasm: 'Well, its *not* your uterus, is it dear? And its *not* your appendix, is it?'

In this case the woman had severe endometriosis and managed

53

to get referred back to a gynaecologist who removed her ovaries (see below). If you are unlucky enough to get a recurrence, this may not be necessary; a six to nine month period of drug treatment may deal with the remaining endometriosis without the need for further surgery. Some women have stayed on low doses of hormones for years to keep their last few symptoms at bay until the natural menopause (see Chapter 3).

If you decide to have a hysterectomy, you will probably be in hospital for a week to ten days and need eight to ten weeks to recover. The operation can be done through an incision in your abdomen or through your vagina (check if you don't know which type is being suggested). An abdominal incision is usually horizontal, below the bikini line, but if you are overweight your gynaecologist may recommend a low vertical incision. A vaginal repair may be done during a vaginal hysterectomy to lift and strengthen support for the vaginal walls.

Some controversy remains about whether or not hysterectomy leads to loss of libido (sex drive), changes in orgasm and depression. Research suggests that depression after hysterectomy may be linked to lack of discussion before the operation and lack of support by family and friends – which seems a natural reaction if you didn't get a proper chance to make your own decision and everyone expected you to get on with it and be right as rain in no time.

Whatever your feelings are, they are important – it is a big decision. You can't change your mind afterwards, in the way that you can if danazol doesn't suit you. The possible benefits of the operation need to be weighed against your endometriosis and your feelings. For some women the relief from pain where other treatments have failed or they did not get on with them has made it all worthwhile.

I took danazol for nine months, struggling with the side effects, but with little help for my symptoms. Things went from bad to worse and a hysterectomy was discussed. I had the operation three weeks later, leaving my remaining tube and ovary. This all happened a year ago and I now feel the best I've felt for years and everyone tells me how well I look and I've loads of energy. I've gained a little weight, work part-time, garden and continue with my yoga. I've just

54

finished painting the bungalow and am learning to swim! Hysterectomy (at 38) was the right decision *for me*.

Some women say freedom from contraception has done wonders for their sex life. A few say their orgasms felt different but didn't disappear as they'd feared.

Other women feel the loss of childbearing and an important part of their bodies, even if they were never desperate to have children.

For me the emotional shock was enormous. . . . I did not really want children, but that did not make it easy for me. Not wanting and being unable are very different things.

I didn't want children, but neither did I want a hysterectomy.

If your endometriosis is mild and you are in your 40s, you may choose to wait until the menopause instead.

I didn't want to lose my uterus which had brought my four children into the world. I was also afraid a hysterectomy would affect my sex life. I asked for another opinion before making up my mind; the second gynaecologist didn't insist that hysterectomy was the only answer and agreed to give me annual check-ups. If I'd had cancer rather than endometriosis, I would have agreed to the op, but my endometriosis pain was manageable and I was willing to wait a year or two until the menopause. I have never regretted my decision.

Finding out more and talking to your doctor, partner and other women about the operation will help you make the decision. Ask for time if you need it. You can contact the Hysterectomy Support Group or the Endometriosis Society's hysterectomy network (see useful addresses on page 151).

REMOVING THE OVARIES

I know the medical profession have differing views on the subject. For instance, the consultant who performed the hysterectomy did not believe in removing the ovaries in someone of my age (I was 36 at the time) whereas Mr X believed that if a woman had severe endometriosis then the ovaries should be removed whatever her age.

Stopping the production of oestrogen by having your ovaries removed (bilateral oophorectomy) may seem the obvious way to deal with endometriosis once and for all, but there is a catch. If you do have your ovaries removed (either at hysterectomy or later), you will start to go through the menopause, whatever your age. This is because the menopause constitutes all the changes your body goes through when your ovaries stop working, either naturally or because they've been removed (surgical menopause). The main symptoms are hot flushes, night sweats and vaginal dryness, although you may experience a variety of other effects (see recommended reading on page 149 for books that give more detail). Long-term problems such as thinning of the vaginal walls (making sex uncomfortable) and osteoporosis (weak brittle bones) can also develop following the menopause and be serious. Doctors are able to stop these changes by giving hormone replacement therapy (HRT).

> My uterus, tubes and ovaries were removed. Symptoms remained but gradually became less and less severe. Six years ago I consulted my doctor about vaginal dryness and was referred for possible HRT. I was given Premarin tablets for two and a half years. The symptoms did not return during treatment and I have not had them since.

> The specialist recommended a hysterectomy which I decided to have. Unfortunately, I had to have both my ovaries out which was a terrifying thought at my age (36). He assured me that with a hormone implant I would feel like a new woman. He was right. I must say that I feel wonderful. I have the implant twice a year. It sounds like a drastic solution, but it is a solution. I feel and think I look younger and it has improved my sex life.

Or you may prefer to investigate alternative approaches (see page 60). If you are deciding whether or not to have your ovaries removed and if you should have HRT or face a surgical menopause, you need to find out as much as possible. Reading around the subjects of the menopause, HRT and alternatives and talking to your doctor, partner and other women who have faced this problem can help you work out your options and what you feel about them (see useful addresses on page 151).

Hormone replacement therapy (HRT)

Hormone replacement therapy (HRT) is designed to replace enough of your natural hormones (oestrogen and progesterone) to prevent the symptoms of menopause. It can be taken continuously until you are ready for the menopause, either as tablets, an implant or in the new skin 'patches' (a small piece of impregnated sticking plaster).

The preparation recommended will depend on several things, apart from your gynaecologist's experience and preference. If you still have your uterus, you must be given a combination of oestrogen and progesterone. This is because one effect of oestrogen is to stimulate growth of the endometrium (see Chapter 1). There is a slightly increased risk of endometrial cancer developing in women given oestrogen 'unopposed' by progesterone, which balances oestrogen's effects and so protects the endometrium. Of course, if you have had a hysterectomy then you won't have an endometrium any more and so can't develop endometrial cancer. In this case you can be given oestrogen on its own or in combination with progesterone or testosterone. There is some evidence that a testosterone implant can improve loss of libido (desire for sex), depression and lethargy associated with the menopause.

HRT is not usually recommended for women with a history of cancer, blood clots or breast cysts. Your doctor may also think twice if you have problems such as diabetes or are a heavy smoker. Talk to your doctor if you are worried about being prescribed HRT, given your medical history.

Oestrogen in HRT has been known to reactivate endometriosis, so you may want to discuss what can be done if this happens. Many GPs are not up to date on this possibility and the debate amongst gynaecologists was reflected in the Endometriosis Society survey. Sixty-one women (8 per cent of all replies) who had had their ovaries out were asked if HRT had been suggested. Just over half had been offered HRT, usually as tablets, whereas a quarter were told they couldn't have HRT because of the risk of reactivating endometriosis. HRT was not suggested to the remaining 25 per cent.

Some doctors suggest starting HRT several months after

SUFFERERS TALK ABOUT HRT

Hormone replacement therapy has its pros and cons and they may look different depending on your age.

Age at op	Advantages	Disadvantages
39	More energy, less tired, mood swings less noticeable, skin not so dry.	Possible recurrence of pain.
38	HRT is very good for hot flushes and other problems if it can be taken.	My endometriosis returned and it took a long time to get back to feeling well again. I don't think I would take it again.
36	General well-being, particularly my energy, skin and hair condition.	Endometriosis may return and no one seems to know the long-term effects of HRT.
36	Protection against osteoporosis. No menopausal symptoms (i.e. flushing). Skin/hair not as oily. Even level of oestrogen with implant (no highs/lows) and can forget about it. No ovarian pain.	Slight risk of disease recurring. Slight worry about side effects (mild headaches). Not suited to everyone.
35	I persevere mainly because of an increased risk of osteoporosis. When I stopped for ten months I had bad sweats and faintness, which I am glad to be free of.	I hate taking tablets and I worry about recurrence. While off HRT I was free of arthritis in my fingers, but as soon as I restarted the pains and swellings came back.

Advantages	_Disadvantags_
31 In my case it is the only answer but I'm afraid it does not work for every-one.	The implants have to be inserted every six months in London. It's the loss of work for one day.
30 In many ways it keeps you feeling your age. After I had my ovaries removed I lost my sexual drive. At 30 this can affect your marriage drastically.	Unfortunately some HRT treatments appear to make endometriosis worse than others. I have tried three types of HRT and at present use Estra-derm 50 patches which seem to suit me.
27 As far as I am concerned HRT keeps me a balanced person. I have no side effects.	Although the implant is not a painful thing to have done, I resent the fact I am dependent on it. Even if I miss my implant by a couple of weeks I can tell the dif-ference in myself.
27 I can't imagine why any-one would not want a controlled low dose of oestrogen to stave off early menopause.	The obvious one of bringing back the endo-metriosis. You must walk a tightrope all the time between too high and too low a dosage. Perhaps if you had your ovaries removed at near menopausal age, you would feel it more natu-ral to go without HRT.

surgery in the hope that this will allow the endometriosis to 'dry up' first.

I had a complete hysterectomy. Two years afer the operation I went on to take HRT which I still take. I have had no recurrence of any previous trouble.

A few doctors recommend a preparation of oestrogen balanced by either progesterone or testosterone to reduce the chances of stimulating any remaining endometriosis. Others argue that the endometriosis is unlikely to come back and, if it does, at least you can stop the HRT for a while or adjust the dose. They may even advocate HRT because they say it is easier to control than the oestrogen produced by the ovaries if you leave them in. Of course, tablets are simpler to change than an implant. If your endometriosis does return or you suffer from side effects (such as nausea, bloatedness, headaches, breast tenderness and mood changes) you may feel better on a different dose or type of HRT.

I started on Premarin 0.625 taken orally but was constantly sick on it. I told my gynaecologist and he prescribed Estraderm – oestrogen is taken in through the skin on a patch you stick on your body, below the waist.

Alternative approaches to HRT
If you agree to a bilateral oophorectomy but decide against HRT, or are unlucky enough to get a recurrence of endometriosis when taking it, you may want to consider alternative ways of alleviating the effects of a surgical menopause. There are many books which describe what can help menopausal symptoms or you may want to try suggestions from other sufferers.

I really did feel ill for ages after my ovaries were removed. Then I embarked on the Ladycare range of vitamins for the menopause. After two weeks the results were dramatic – no flushes! I felt so much better, stronger and not so depressed.

I took HRT for six weeks and endometriosis returned. I heard on a radio programme that royal jelly could be used for problems of the menopause. I gave it a try and it works very well. I take it with evening primrose oil. (See Chapter 5.)

I took *Agnus castus* (see Chapter 5) as a replacement for HRT – burning feeling in body and headaches improved. I did not expect it to clear symptoms, but it did!

I found that evening primrose oil relieves hot flushes and makes me feel more comfortable. This took effect after two months. Symptoms returned after I stopped taking it.

If your vagina gets dry, your doctor can prescribe vaginal oestrogen creams which can help enormously. Do not be tempted to use them as a lubricant during sex as they can be absorbed through your partner's skin too! A little vitamin E oil carefully rubbed into the vagina is an alternative to oestrogen cream.

Osteoporosis

Osteoporosis is a very common problem in women after the menopause because lack of oestrogen in some way seems to allow the calcium content of bone to be reduced, with the result that your skeleton becomes brittle and more likely to break. Many older women develop bent backs (and may actually shrink in height) because weak vertebrae in their spines become compressed and crumble. The Osteoporosis Society (see Useful Addresses on page 152) recommends ways of preventing this, including increasing calcium in your diet and regular exercise, although recent studies suggest that extra calcium may not be as protective as originally hoped. HRT is still the best way to prevent osteoporosis, but treatments based on other hormones such as calcitonin (which 'pushes' calcium from the blood into the bones) are being developed which may help if you can't take HRT.

LASER LAPAROSCOPY

A laser produces a high-energy beam of light that can be very accurately controlled (e.g. using mirrors) so that, for example, it is possible to cut grooves in a human hair to a specified depth. The ability to destroy tissue in a precise place without damage to the surrounding area makes the laser an increasingly popular surgical tool. The tissue is sealed as the laser cuts, so there is little bleeding, and the area heals very fast and returns to its normal function without being obstructed by adhesions or fibrosis.

Lasers adapted for use down a laparoscope (laser laparoscopy) can avoid the need for major surgery. This has obvious advantages for the patient, but does make life much more difficult for the gynaecologist. According to one surgeon, inexperienced doctors tend to feel that using a very powerful tool in a confined space where they can only see and feel indirectly is a bit like '*Star Wars* in the pelvis'! Using more than one puncture (you may have two or three tiny scars) helps improve visibility and removal of debris (and smoke!). With experience, a laser can be used to cut up cysts (which are drained and extracted through the laparoscope) or to destroy endometriosis near very delicate areas such as the ureter or bowel. Adding a video camera to the system allows the surgeon to record the operation and endometriosis sites for future reference.

Initial research suggests that endometriosis doesn't come back at sites where it has been treated, but in up to 50 per cent of cases it recurs at different sites – possibly ones the surgeon could not see at the time (remember that endometriosis may only be visible in its later stages). The surgeon may then recommend a course of hormone tablets to deal with remaining endometriosis; alternatively, you may want to try and get pregnant straight after the surgery.

Lasers can also be used to separate adhesions, which may in themselves cause more problems than endometriosis, but women who have adhesions fixing their uterus against the bowel, or similar problems, cannot expect too much. Most surgeons will not risk damaging the bowel in an attempt to free scar tissue, although techniques are improving all the time. Research should be available before long which compares laser surgery with other treatments for endometriosis.

Angela was diagnosed when a chocolate cyst on her left ovary ruptured. She had a laparotomy and 'all the painful after-effects of such surgery'. Four months later, a scan revealed another cyst in the same place. She considered whether or not to have surgery again.

I decided to have the cyst removed whilst it was still fairly small as I could not bear the thought, or pain, of another rupture, and a bit of detective work led me to laser surgery.

I was admitted as a day case. The surgery took just 90 minutes (even though I have severe endometriosis) and I was able to leave the hospital at 6 pm the same day. The whole experience was a lot less traumatic than previously. The laser was inserted through a half-inch cut in my abdomen, the adhesions burnt off, the cyst drained and burnt off as much as possible. Recuperation was a lot quicker than conventional surgery. I did suffer some pain for two weeks afterwards (where my cyst had been), but since then I have been pain free. The only reminder of the operation is a small scar. I am not receiving any hormone treatment for the condition and have instead been seeing a homoeopath, and am responding very well to this treatment.

Nicola also had severe endometriosis and problems with recurrent chocolate cysts.

My endometriosis was diagnosed and I had my left ovary and Fallopian tube removed. My main symptoms were severe pain, lethargy, heavy bleeding and severe PMT. Six years later (at 40) I was advised to have a total hysterectomy; my uterus was totally fixed and I had a large cyst in the pouch of Douglas. I was devastated. My GP was very supportive and tried to help me to come to terms with the situation psychologically. With my GP's and gynaecologist's approval, I went to see a consultant who agreed to perform laser surgery. I had no discomfort immediately after surgery – not even from the three small incisions in my abdomen where the instruments went in. After a few days I did have severe pain before defaecation, which eventually settled down. I also had some side effects from the anaesthetic. I saw my usual gynaecologist six months later and he was very impressed with the improvement – my uterus is free again. As my endometriosis is still active I may have to have further laser surgery in the future. Meanwhile, my periods are far less severe and I have been able to avoid having a total hysterectomy and its complications at least for some time.

5

ALTERNATIVE AND COMPLEMENTARY APPROACHES

This chapter is based on the experiences of endometriosis sufferers who have found help using different approaches to the orthodox treatments described in Chapters 3 and 4. Many have been able to relieve their symptoms; others feel they have found a complete cure. Sufferers often try alternative medicine when they feel drugs and surgery have not helped, but some have found therapies complementary to the treatment they are receiving.

A wide range of supplements, remedies and alternative approaches are briefly described. Do turn to the recommended reading and useful addresses lists if you want to investigate anything in more detail or contact a practitioner. Do not expect immediate results; many comments show that you need to allow at least a month or two before you give up. In some cases, you may find symptoms get worse initially. Alternative practitioners – like doctors – do not necessarily agree on the best approach to endometriosis, but this chapter will give you a starting point.

DO THEY WORK?

Many people report benefits from alternative approaches but there have been very few studies of their effectiveness (partly because of lack of research monies). A good test would be to compare the medicine with an inactive product (placebo) in a double-blind placebo-controlled trial. Unmarked pills are given, so neither researchers nor volunteers (double-blind) know who received what until afterwards. These sort of trials are important because they allow for the 'placebo effect'; research shows one would expect up to 30 per cent of patients taking the inactive pill to report improvements, so anything that is active should have even better results. No one knows why the placebo effect occurs but it may be to do with people's expectations that any treatment will help – an example of mind over matter.

Of course, few treatments, even those described in Chapters 3 and 4, have been tested in this way. Clinical trials for drugs tend to compare drugs with each other rather than with a placebo, simply because of the ethical problems of giving a patient inactive pills when this may not be in her best interests. Alternative practitioners will feel a similar obligation to treat someone with something they believe will help rather than do research on her. And there are ethical and practical problems in testing surgery in this way – surgeons cannot be blind to what they are doing, and cannot justify opening one patient up and treating her and opening another up and not treating her for the sake of comparison. All this means the debate about what has been proven to be effective – whether orthodox or alternative – is complicated and that you will need to judge studies and individual experiences in this light. On the other hand, if you find something that works, you might not be too worried about whether or not it is the placebo effect as long as it lasts.

VITAMINS, MINERALS, OILS AND EXTRACTS

Sufferers have found various supplements relieve complaints such as premenstrual syndrome (PMS) and pain (also see Chapter 9). Supplements are expensive so you may prefer to use natural food sources wherever possible.

Vitamin B6 and vitamin B complex
In the early 1970s researchers reported the successful use of vitamin B6 to combat depression in women on the pill. More recent studies have demonstrated significant improvements in premenstrual symptoms in 50–60 per cent of patients on 80–100 mg per day. Vitamin B6 is now a popular home remedy for PMS and many GPs prescribe it.

The reasons why vitamin B6 should help PMS are still poorly

66

understood, but it appears to be important in the production of certain substances influencing the pituitary gland (and hence the menstrual cycle) and the production of other chemicals thought to regulate mood. Many endometriosis sufferers have found vitamin B6 helps PMS symptoms such as irritability and bloatedness which they report throughout the month, while others have found that it reduces side effects of hormone treatment, especially tiredness and depression.

The starting dose recommended for PMS is 50 mg of vitamin B6 twice a day with meals, increasing the dose if necessary. Megadosing (500 mg/day or more) in the USA highlighted the danger of nervous disorders which develop when you take too much vitamin B6. Up to 200 mg/day is said to be safe, although the maximum dose can cause stomach upsets. In addition to vitamin B6, 25–50 mg of vitamin B complex is often recommended, particularly if you are under a lot of stress, have problems eating a balanced diet or suffer from poor absorption, but you must note the dose of vitamin B6 in the complex tablet so you do not take too much altogether.

Brewer's yeast, wheatgerm, cabbage and eggs are amongst good sources of vitamin B6.

Evening primrose oil (EPO)

The American Indians used evening primrose oil (EPO) for asthma and skin disorders, but it has recently become popular for premenstrual symptoms. An open study (i.e. not blind) showed that 62 per cent of women with PMS, who had not responded to other treatments, showed an improvement with EPO (i.e. better than would be expected, taking into account the placebo effect). Out of 36 women who suffered very tender breasts, 26 found this symptom improved dramatically, especially if they also stopped drinking tea and coffee.

Evening primrose oil is an important source of gamma-linolenic acid (GLA) which probably accounts for its effectiveness. GLA is an essential fatty acid which helps the body produce a hormone-like chemical called prostaglandin E_1 (PGE_1 for short). PGE_1 regulates several body functions thought to be involved in the development of PMS. There is also evidence that zinc, magnesium, vitamin C, niacin and vitamin B6 are needed as part of this process – experience at a London hospital suggests that taking these as supplements, or making the appropriate dietary improvements, increases the effectiveness of evening primrose oil for PMS, although a proper trial has not been done yet. Evening primrose oil also blocks overproduction of leukotrines, substances thought to be involved in certain types of pain which are not amenable to painkillers such as aspirin (which block prostaglandins, see Chapter 9).

More importantly in this context, endometriosis sufferers have also found evening primrose oil helpful, and trials are now underway testing it as a way of relieving symptoms rather than reducing visible endometriosis.

Mood swings – improved within a month; adhesion pain – improved within two months; period cramps – slightly better.

Severe abdominal pain, difficulty in walking, dryness in vagina, all relieved within ten days of starting EPO.

I have been taking EPO for 18 months. I start on the 10th day of my cycle (3 or 4 × 500 mg daily). I no longer feel extreme tiredness and lethargy (some months I used to be too tired to go to work and had no energy for a social life). I used to have spots, cold sores and a very swollen stomach. My complexion is much healthier and friends keep remarking on how well I am looking. My periods used to be heavy, with painful bowel movements (endometriosis in bowel). I still have some pain, but nothing I cannot cope with, and only a faint show of bleeding from bowel. My GP was sceptical at first but he has since informed me that a local hospital had good results using EPO for breast cysts, and he now admits it could possibly have the same sort of effect with endometriosis. There have been months when I just haven't been able to afford EPO and all my past symptoms return within a few weeks. The only criticism I have is that my bust has grown from 34 to 36 inches, but that is a very small price to pay!

Sufferers have also found that evening primrose oil helps side effects of hormone treatments.

Side effects from danazol, e.g. muscle spasms and pains, vanished completely with EPO but returned during the week's trial break I took.

At present I take 800 mg/day of danazol and find EPO a great help in keeping the side effects at bay.

Look out for other preparations containing GLA, e.g. borage seed oil or glanolin from blackcurrant seeds. Cold-pressed safflower oil (10 ml twice daily) can be a cheaper way of taking GLA. Try a local healthfood shop.

Vitamin E

Vitamin E is recommended by some to help prevent thick scar formation and to maintain a healthy skin. Sufferers report that 600–1,000 international units (iu) per day helps pain which they associate with their adhesions. Vitamin E is also advised if you have fertility problems, on the basis that animals with vitamin E deficiency lose their fertility. However if you have high blood pressure and are on anticoagulent drugs, check with your doctor before taking vitamin E.

There is some debate about whether vitamin E affects oestrogen levels. Some argue that it regulates oestrogen and is beneficial; others warn that vitamin E may not be advisable if you have had your ovaries removed and do not want to run the risk of reactivating endometriosis. You will need to read round this subject before making up your mind (see recommended reading).

Vitamin E is found in green vegetables, wholegrain cereals, soya beans and eggs.

Vitamin C

Vitamin C can help if you suffer from heavy bleeding; it strengthens blood-vessel walls and aids absorption of iron (a vital constituent of red blood cells), particularly if taken with bioflavonoids (for a time these were known as vitamin P). It can also promote healing after surgery. Some sufferers strongly recommend it for help with pain.

When I feel the inflammation from endometriosis increasing I step up my intake of vitamin C to 4–5 grams daily and within 24 hours there is a reduction in the inflammatory pain.

Selenium

Selenium is a trace element, i.e. it is essential for good health although only minute amounts are needed in the diet. Several animal studies have shown that selenium has useful anti-inflammatory effects and can improve the immune system, which could account for the benefits people report from taking it. For example, a Russian study on rabbits suggests that a combination of selenium and vitamin E leads to more antibody production in response to a vaccine than does selenium on its own, while open studies on patients indicate that selenium can help inflammation in rheumatic disease, and endometriosis sufferers report very positive results with symptoms of pain (although it may need time to act).

> There has been a steady improvement in pain over the past four months. I shall take selenium for the rest of my life quite happily and can hardly believe how much benefit I have had from it – in fact every bit as much improvement as when on danazol or Duphaston, which I was prescribed over the previous four years and which had such bad side effects.

> My symptoms diminished but danazol had a lot of side effects. As soon as I stopped taking it, the pain and diarrhoea started again. I was reluctant to have the remaining ovary removed and the consultant was reluctant to operate. However, after four months on selenium the pain is much relieved, the diarrhoea has stopped and I feel very much better in myself. The consultant is delighted. He is doing research into endometriosis and has asked me to send him any literature on selenium.

> Both the nagging pain on my right side and rundown feeling were much better after two to three weeks, and I feel much more able to cope with things.

Selenium is available commercially in several forms. Selenium ACE is based on yeast cultured with selenium, combined with vitamins A, C and E. Some authors suggest that a yeast (organic) base makes the selenium more effective (increases its bioavailability). If you are allergic to yeast or on an anti-candida diet (see page 82), selenium is available without yeast (check the label carefully). One or two side effects reported may be caused by a yeast base rather than the selenium itself.

70

I have had good results from selenium, but have had to give it up as it gives me fiendish indigestion.

The dose of selenium ACE recommended by the makers is a capsule a day (i.e. 100 micrograms (µg) selenium), but endometriosis sufferers have used three times this dose without ill-effects. Onions and garlic, broccoli, tomatoes, wheatgerm and tuna are good sources of selenium.

Magnesium

Magnesium is important in the metabolism of linoleic acid (another of the essential fatty acids) and the prevention of PMS. Magnesium levels are much lower than normal in red blood cells of women with premenstrual syndrome, and were doubled after four weeks of 2×100 mg/day vitamin B6. Magnesium is also necessary for calcium and vitamin C metabolism.

Try a supplement of 300–400 mg/day (not to be taken after meals), or eating plenty of green leafy vegetables, grapefruit, figs, apples, almonds, nuts and seeds in your diet. You will be getting more magnesium if you live in a hard water area. Avoid diet drinks which contain phosphorus, which tends to block absorption of magnesium.

Taking magnesium with calcium in supplements such as dolomite, aids the absorption of both minerals (see below).

Calcium

Painful muscle spasms and period cramps have been attributed to low blood calcium levels occurring at the end of the menstrual cycle. Some sufferers have found a calcium preparation such as dolomite helps painful periods and joint pains associated with endometriosis.

I had joint pains in my knees for many years prior to dolomite and haven't had them since. I recommend six tablets daily.

Dairy products are well-known for their calcium content, but there are other ways of getting what you need without the fat in milk – dried beans, green vegetables, peanuts, walnuts, sunflower seeds and sardines are also good sources.

Zinc

Zinc is another mineral thought to be valuable in treatment of premenstrual syndrome, which is common amongst women with endometriosis. It also has other relevant benefits such as promoting healing and fertility. There are various zinc testers on the market which will help you find out if you are deficient. The recommended dose is 15–25 mg/day.

Good foods for zinc are eggs, herrings, oysters, wheatgerm, seeds and nuts. Avoid a lot of bran, which is said to prevent absorption.

Supplement 'cocktails'

Selecting what might help you from the above may be a bit daunting. The experiences of women writing in to the Endometriosis Society suggest that the following daily 'cocktail' of vitamins can be very helpful, either to help symptoms or to relieve the side effects of drug treatment.

- Up to 150 mg vitamin B6 with 50 mg vitamin B complex.
- 1–2 g vitamin C.
- 200–1,000 iu vitamin E.
- Up to 20,000 iu vitamin A.
- 6 tablets dolomite (calcium/magnesium).
- 10–30 mg zinc.
- 1 multivitamin/multimineral tablet.

Since last October I have been taking vitamin B6, 500 mg EPO and a good multivitamin daily. I feel a new woman and no longer have the feeling of complete exhaustion all the time.

Since beginning danazol in May I have been taking one multivitamin, 1 g vitamin C, 100 mg vitamin B6 with B complex, two selenium ACE daily. I believe that these helped to fight off the negative effects of danazol – I was out of vitamins for a number of weeks and there was a huge difference in my levels of energy.

Along with Primolut N (5 mg/daily) and selenium ACE (three tabs daily) I take many other vitamins which I believe all contribute to my much improved state of health.

I was 35 when I realised that conventional medicine alone was not going to be the answer to my future health. Armed with Mega B100, vitaman C, vitamin E, wild yam (a herbal anti-spasmodic) and the peppermint pill, plus a little fibregel, I was out of pain for the first time in years and able to eat almost anything painlessly.

You may prefer to try supplements one at a time instead, so you get an idea of what works for you – and avoid the expense of what does not. Or you can seek advice from an alternative practitioner who specialises in nutritional or vitamin therapies.

BIOCHEMIC TISSUE SALTS

I have suffered from insomnia and 'nervous tension' for many years. Kali Phos makes me sleep well, relax, feel calmer and more able to cope.

The Schussler system of biochemic medicine identifies 12 salts responsible for the way the body functions. Any problems are seen as an imbalance in one or more of these salts. Tissue salts are often prescribed by homoeopaths, but you can also try them yourself as they are available in health shops. You may find the following useful for certain problems:

- Kali Phos   for PMT and depression
- Calc Phos   for light periods
- Kali Phos, Silica   for heavy periods
- Nat Mur or Nat Sulph   for fluid retention
- Mag Phos   for painful periods
- Combination S salts   for menstrual nausea

The usual method of taking them is to dissolve them on your tongue with nothing to eat or drink and no teeth-cleaning in the next hour. Guidelines on dose are given on the container.

HERBAL MEDICINE

Herbs can be used in home remedies for various complaints as well as part of a regime prescribed by a herbalist. Some simple self-help methods are recommended for endometriosis sufferers by the Secretary of the National Institute of Medical Herbalists in the box on page 74.

Treatment by a qualified herbalist can be very helpful for pain. The prescription recommended will depend on your case, but the tinctures (solutions of herbs) are bound to have lovely names, as well as offering help! A list of practitioners can be obtained from the National Institute of Medical Herbalists (see useful addresses).

SELF-HELP WITH HERBS

Pain	See page 135.
Tiredness, depression, irritability	Try herb teas to replace ordinary tea and coffee – peppermint or rosemary will invigorate, chamomile and limeflower will soothe and relax.
Tired headache	Try a mixture of essential oils of peppermint and lavender, one drop smeared on to the forehead (take care not to get it in the eyes).
Bladder pain, irritable bladder (where there is no infection)	Try meadowsweet tea, made like ordinary tea – one cupful (without milk) four times a day or as required. One batch can be prepared and kept in a flask or reheated, but a fresh batch should be made daily.
Digestive problems	Try ginger (see page 135). This can be used for flatulence or for colicky pains. Two slippery elm tablets chewed between meals can soothe – slippery elm has a healing action and is well tolerated. It can also counteract irritation of the stomach caused by some drugs.

I took tinctures of thyme, licorice black coloch, vitex, St Johnswort, motherwort and nettle – 15 drops on empty stomach three times a day. My healer also suggested hot and cold water treatments each day on my abdomen and a loose vegetarian diet involving raw veg and nuts. So far I have had two totally pain-free periods.

At present I am taking violet leaf tea three times a day. Ugh! After suffering black/brown periods for 16 months I have had the first (three day only – wow) red-blood period. Violet leaves are an exfoliant and wash out everything in the wrong place.

My menopause symptoms are controlled by herbal medicine. Unless something untoward is going on, I feel randy most of the time and I control my vaginal dryness with oestrogen creams. I have to have an extremely good diet otherwise things go haywire. Unless I look at the stress in my life and try and control it, symptoms return with a vengeance.

Vitex agnus castus

Agnus castus is a herb native to the Mediterranean, first recommended by the Egyptians for sexual disorders in women long before anyone knew about hormone imbalances. It is also known as chaste tree, reputedly because nuns used it to suppress sexual urges.

Research in Sweden suggests that *Agnus castus* affects hormones produced by the pituitary gland. Alternative practitioners recommend it for a variety of menstrual problems, including infertility. It is also said to be a mild antidepressant. Endometriosis sufferers have found it useful for various symptoms.

Mood changes and cycle pain much improved.

Greatly improved mood swings, depression and PMT.

Occasionally, though, people react badly to it.

Did try taking *Agnus castus* but it gave me a headache, diarrhoea and made me feel dizzy, so I stopped taking them.

Agnus castus should NOT be used at the same time as hormone treatments.

75

Agnus castus is available commercially as an extract (it may be called agnolyt) or tablets. You may need to take it for several months until symptoms subside; then take it for a few further weeks. Some herbalists feel that you should only use *Agnus castus* under guidance.

HOMOEOPATHY

You might be forgiven for confusing herbal medicine and homoeopathy because the latter also uses remedies with exotic sounding names. However, homoeopathy is based on certain principles rather than certain medicines.

Homoeopathic principles were formulated 200 years ago by Samuel Hahnemann, a German physician who was disillusioned with 18th-century medicine which he saw as ineffective, with harmful, even lethal, side effects. He based his principles on years of methodical work testing his ideas.

One of the most important principles is the 'law of similars' – that the substance to cure symptoms is the one which causes temporary symptoms in healthy people. There are around 6,000 substances which qualify as homoeopathic remedies. Another principle dictates they should be prepared through a careful series of dilutions and shaking. Apart from making the solution harmless, this process is said to allow the substance to change from inert to dynamic; then it is seen more as an energy stimulating an organ's own self-healing powers. Many scientists argue that the solutions are so dilute that the original substance cannot still exist in it, but research published in the respected journal *Nature* (1988) suggests that dilution and shaking somehow 'imprints' the substance on water molecules long after the substance has been diluted out. So the debate is likely to continue.

Homoeopathic remedies can lead to symptoms worsening initially; indeed practitioners often expect to take a sufferer through past illness, and a resurgence is seen as bringing out deeper levels of complaint for treatment. This process is described by several endometriosis sufferers who found homoeopathy very helpful.

My very first remedy produced a terrible aggravation of symptoms, i.e. flooding and pain. However, my second remedy worked like a miracle and I had my first virtually painless and light period in years. From that point things began to improve. I suppose, honestly, I feel it has taken me four years of treatment before I was free of any endometriosis symptoms, and throughout those years homoeopathy has helped me to re-evaluate my life and ideals. It has also kindled a strong interest which I am pursuing on a full-time course in homoeopathy.

In desperation I went to a homoeopath. The treatment, sceptically begun, was dramatic. The remedy almost immediately made me iller than I had ever been, for about seven to ten days, but once through this phase I got better and better and was virtually symptom-free for three months. Then it began to get really interesting – my symptoms returned, but in a changed form. Apparently the remedy 'bumped into' glandular fever which I had when I was 16! My homoeopath treated the glandular fever and I have been getting steadily better. She is still working through the 'sludge' of past ailments, but I feel better than I have done for years. It has been difficult at times to stick with it, as 're-living' symptoms is far from pleasant, but infinitely preferable to a bottle of tranquillisers!

Within six weeks a very depressed weepy, moody and very unhappy person changed. I started to have energy, to live and enjoy life. The pain started to go and after a year I was feeling strong and very well. I still have little relapses when I am under a lot of stress and have allowed myself to become run down. I think the hardest part of alternative medicine was realising it works – its approach and theory is so different to mainstream medicine that I found it difficult to trust.

My first session was one hour devoted to me as a whole person, my history of health and illness, emotional behaviour and lifestyle. I came away with a changing perspective. I began to consider that it might be inevitable that I would develop a chronic illness because I had persistently failed to rest or ask for support during prolonged periods of stress, until I became ill. A month after this, all symptoms of endometriosis returned, almost as severely as ever. I continued with homoeopathy. My menstrual flow responded quickly to treatment (in my case pulsatilla). I am now five months pregnant and feel well and optimistic.

The third homoeopathic principle is to treat an individual's experience of symptoms rather than seeing them as part of an underlying disease.

For a reliable practitioner consult the Register of Homoeopaths available from the Society of Homoeopaths (see useful addresses).

A MACROBIOTIC DIET

A macrobiotic diet is based on eating whole, unrefined foods – no meat, refined sugar or dairy products. Cereal grains, beans, vegetables, fruits, seeds and seaweed, plus some fish and seafood are the staples. Those with a sweet tooth will be reassured by delicious desserts made with grain-based sweeteners (barley malt and rice syrup).

I originally investigated the macrobiotic diet because from all reports it seemed to be the best way of improving the immune system and healing myself naturally without the use of drugs or surgery. My problems, apart from moderate endometriosis, included a small ovarian cyst, a fibroid and malfunctioning tube, so my chances of getting pregnant were pretty slim. In addition, I had low back pain, rectal cramp, pain during intercourse and a persistent leg pain, plus the unpleasant mental symptoms of depression and anxiety. After 20 months of adhering strictly to the diet, I brought my endometriosis under control and found myself pregnant (at 41!). The doctors, needless to say, were amazed!

The dietary programme is restrictive but the cooking is straightforward and cookery classes are available at various macrobiotic centres throughout the country. Patience and determination are needed, but the results can be spectactular!

CANDIDA ALBICANS

American physicians interested in *Candida albicans* noticed that symptoms of endometriosis often improved with anti-

A ROUGH GUIDE TO CANDIDIASIS

An alternative practitioner specialising in candida usually does an allergy test for yeast based on muscle function. Saying yes to many of these questions *may* indicate that you have a candida problem.

Drug usage

- Have you had lengthy, or repeated, courses of antibiotics (longer than eight weeks on end, or more than four short courses in one year)?
- Have you been treated for acne with antibiotics for more than one month continuously?
- Have you had steroid (hormonal) treatment?
- Have you had contraceptive medication for a year or more?
- Have you been pregnant more than once (this alters the hormonal balance in favour of candida)?
- Have you had a course of immunosuppressive drugs?

Symptoms

- Have you had persistent, or recurrent, cystitis, vaginitis, urethritis?
- Have you a history of pelvic inflammatory disease or endometriosis?
- Have you had recurrent thrush (oral or vaginal)?
- Have you had athlete's foot, or other fungal infections on the hands, nails, etc?
- Are you severely affected by exposure to fumes, pollutants, perfumes, etc?
- Do you have a variety of allergies?
- Do you suffer from abdominal bloating, distension and diarrhoea or constipation?
- Do you suffer from premenstrual syndrome?
- Are you lethargic, depressed, unnaturally fatigued?
- Do you suffer from poor memory or feelings of unreality?
- Do you crave sweet foods, bread or alcohol?
- Do you have unaccounted-for aches and pains?
- Do you have vaginal discharge and/or menstrual cramps?
- Do you suffer from lack of sexual desire?
- Do you frequently have spots before your eyes?

(From 'Your body's unwelcome guests' by Leon Chaitow, *Alternative Medicine Today*) candida treatment. *Candida albicans* is a microscopic organism related to the common yeasts used to make bread or alcohol. It takes up residence in the gut (from the mouth through to the anus), vagina and urethra soon after you are born. If you have had thrush, then you know it well – it's caused by the same organism.

Normally, your body keeps colonies of candida under control but an upset in body chemistry or a weakened immune system can lead to growth getting out of hand, causing problems. For example, you may have noticed that you get thrush more frequently when you are on the pill or after taking antibiotics. Drugs which suppress the immune system can have a similar effect. Deficiencies in zinc, linoleic acid and vitamins B6 and C are also said to be associated with the proliferation of candida. People who are heavy smokers, drink a lot of tea and coffee and are under prolonged stress are likely to have a candida problem.

Thrush may be the most familiar sign of unchecked candida growth (candidiasis), but several authors have suggested that the yeast can also get into the bloodstream, causing a whole range of other symptoms. In this case they argue that candidiasis should be regarded as a systemic disease (i.e. affecting the body as a whole) and predict that problems will return if treatment is limited to localised measures such as use of vaginal creams/pessaries. No one knows whether systemic candida causes endometriosis or a weak immune system means you are likely to have both. Several sufferers have treated candidiasis themselves: others prefer to consult a practitioner (write to Endometriosis Society or Candida Albicans Advice Group for details). This can be done while you are taking hormone treatments.

Treatment for candida
The treatment recommended by practitioners specialising in candidiasis has three stages: anti-fungal remedies which kill candida; supplements to restore 'friendly' bacteria in the bowel; and an anti-candida diet which discourages its regrowth, with vitamins and minerals to strengthen the immune system.

Medically qualified alternative practitioners can prescribe the fungicide Nystatin. The powder is preferable if you are on an anti-candida diet (see page 82) since the pills are sugar-coated. The powder can also be mixed with water and used as a mouthwash to treat or prevent oral thrush, before being swallowed. Other anti-fungal substances are available commercially.

- Caprylic acid – very effective fungicide derived from coconut oil.
- Pau d'arco tea – derived from the bark of an Argentinian tree and containing lapachol which acts as a fungicide. Other names include tahhebo, lapacho and ipe roxo. Pau d'arco teabags are available, or it can be taken in capsules or as a herbal extract.
- Organic garlic – good anti-fungal agent. Take it as capsules if you prefer (e.g. kyolic).
- Chlorophyll – toxic to candida. Available as a supplement.
- Homoeopathic remedy – your homoeopath may prescribe a dilution of candida or health shops may stock Nelson's candida dilution.

Many of the fungicides described above will destroy 'friendly' bowel bacteria as well, which you will need to replace. You may be surprised to learn you could have as much as 3–5 lb of bacteria to replace, but once colonies are re-started they should grow back again quite happily. Practitioners often recommend that you begin with *Lactobacillus bifido*, especially if you were not breastfed (a good source of this bacteria originally). Preparations include Vitaplex and Probion Bifidus. Then use Superdophilus, a very good source of *Lactobacillus acidophilus* (if you are allergic to milk use Primedophilus). Taking biotin (a B vitamin) is also said to be important because it stops candida converting into its more destructive form. Oleic acid (occurs in olive oil) also has this effect, so 300 micrograms of biotin are recommended three times a day with two tablespoons of olive oil. Restoring the balance can take one to six months depending on the severity of symptoms.

Anti-candida diet

The anti-candida diet is designed to starve existing candida and prevent its regrowth. It is seen as an essential step because you cannot expect to control candida while you continue to eat foods which contain sugar and yeast and so encourage its growth. Various books (see recommended reading) describe the diet in detail and cookery books will help you adjust your habits. There are still many things you can eat, such as fruit and vegetables, wholemeal cereals, certain grains, fish, eggs and organic meat.

Vitamins and mineral supplements are recommended to increase mucous linings (e.g. in the gut and vagina) to prevent candida passing into the bloodstream. They are also intended to strengthen the immune system so your body is better able to control candida colonies. Megadoses are recommended for therapy which are then reduced to maintenance doses, but you should consult a practitioner for advice, since people have different needs.

Drastic as treating candida sounds, some sufferers have had good results.

It is early days, but already the anti-candida regime has brought about great improvements. The first and most obvious change was loss of weight. Constant visits to the loo shed 17 lb of fluid in as many days! I found I had so much energy I drove my husband to distraction! I both looked and felt so much better. So far as the endometriosis is concerned, I am keeping my fingers crossed but my last two periods have been pain-free – altogether a miracle!

And several years later she writes:

I have now been pain-free for over three years. Periods are mostly clear and bright for approximately three days and often arrive without any prior warning whatsoever. I am on maintenance doses of vitamins which suit me, but no longer take beta carotene. I loosely observe the diet, although I still avoid bread and yeast foods generally. My main weakness is sugary foods and I do not always exert the self-discipline I should!

Dr X diagnosed candida and zinc deficiency by energy contact or muscle testing. She prescribed a yeast-and-sugar-free diet; apart from the obvious I had to cut out cheese, mushrooms, alcohol, chocolate, coffee and tea. I also had to take zinc orotate 100 mg three times a day. Miraculously, within five days my usual fuzzy head cleared and the pains in my stomach subsided. My energy level was about the same – tiring easily and needing a good eight hours at night and a cat nap during the day. After about 11 months on the diet, which after the initial shock I became quite used to (and with careful selection could manage to eat out on occasionally), Dr D said the candida was clear and I could introduce sugars again. I had lost 1½ stone, which was excess anyway. One tip worth mentioning about cooking is to introduce a variety of fresh or dried herbs to make the food more interesting.

6

ENDOMETRIOSIS AND INFERTILITY

by Caroline Hawkridge and Dr Stephen Kennedy

For me the worst thing was not being able to have a baby. This has been the biggest disappointment in my life causing tremendous emotional distress. However, this is now behind me and I have learnt to come to terms with the situation, although there are times when I feel a bit down.

If you have just been diagnosed as having endometriosis and want to know if you will be able to have children, statistics and medical opinions are not easy to juggle. If you have a history of infertility you will want to know if treating your endometriosis will give you a better chance of conceiving.

This chapter will not provide all the answers, but it explains ways in which endometriosis could cause infertility and it discusses the merits of treatment options currently available. It also touches on sufferers' feelings about infertility and their experience of techniques such as in vitro fertilisation (IVF) and gamete intra-Fallopian transfer (GIFT). Several good books discuss being infertile in more detail (see recommended reading), or it may help you to get in touch with others through the Endometriosis Society or National Association for the Childless (see useful addresses).

UNDERSTANDING THE POSSIBLE LINK

Endometriosis is associated with infertility – 30–70 per cent of women investigated for infertility are found to have endometriosis, and 30–40 per cent of sufferers cannot conceive. However, these figures do not necessarily mean that endometriosis *causes* infertility. This issue is still hotly debated, although most of the controversy is about whether mild endometriosis causes infertility; there is little argument about severe endometriosis.

Severe endometriosis destroys normal pelvic anatomy and so it is easy to see why it could cause infertility. A Fallopian tube stuck down by adhesions cannot pick up an egg and an egg cannot easily be released from an ovary containing large endometriotic (chocolate) cysts. This does not imply that you cannot become pregnant or there are no treatments which may help if you have severe endometriosis; pregnancy is possible, but it is best to be realistic about the problems that severe endometriosis causes and how they could prevent fertility. No one knows why endometriosis should become severe in some women and not others.

Mild endometriosis is defined as implants scattered on the peritoneum, without chocolate cysts or anatomical distortions caused by adhesions. So why should mild endometriosis cause infertility – if at all? Do some women who are infertile happen, coincidentally, to have endometriosis as well, just as they may have blue eyes? Endometriosis is quite common, so some infertile women could have endometriosis by chance; likewise infertility is common, so some endometriosis sufferers may be infertile by chance.

This is an important question, not only from a scientific point of view; it would obviously be wrong to expect a woman to take drugs with potentially unpleasant side effects for a condition not actually contributing to her infertility, unless there were other problems such as pain which the drugs might ease. However, it is quite common for women suffering from infertility who are diagnosed as having endometriosis to have no symptoms.

Research into mild endometriosis as a possible cause of infertility has concentrated on three main areas – ovarian function, sperm transport and the immunology of endometriosis. These are complicated subjects in their own right; if you wish to pursue them, they are covered in more (rather technical) detail in medical texts on endometriosis (see recommended reading on page 149).

Ovarian function

A few women with mild endometriosis are anovulatory (they do not ovulate spontaneously), but so are many infertile women without endometriosis. However, treatment with drugs like Clomid, designed to make you ovulate, tend not to be successful in women with endometriosis until the disease itself is treated.

Luteinised unruptured follicle syndrome (LUFS) is said to be more common in women with endometriosis. This means that a follicle responds to the surge of luteinising hormone (LH) during the menstrual cycle (see Chapter 1) by preparing itself for ovulation, but fails to rupture; and of course, if the egg is not released conception cannot occur. Fertility measurements such as a mid-cycle body temperature rise and elevated progesterone levels in the second half of the cycle will suggest ovulation has occurred, but be misleading because the egg is still trapped inside the follicle. Diagnosis can only be made by looking for the absence of a stigma (the hole made in the follicle by the release of the egg) during a laparoscopy or by repeated ultrasound measurements of follicle diameter – normally the follicle shrinks after ovulation, but this does not occur in women with LUFS. So many studies have reported a strong association between LUFS and endometriosis that some researchers have even suggested that LUFS is the cause of endometriosis, rather than the converse.

Another reason why women with mild endometriosis may be infertile is that the corpus luteum (see Chapter 1) may not produce enough progesterone in the second half of the menstrual cycle, known as the luteal phase. This leads to short menstrual cycles and may mean that a fertilised egg cannot implant properly.

Sperm transport

Assuming your partner has enough sperm, they still have to reach the egg if conception is going to take place. Apart from their ability to 'swim', they are helped along by the Fallopian tube's muscular contractions. The strength of these contractions is influenced by many factors, including chemicals called prostaglandins which are produced by many tissues, including patches of endometriosis. Prostaglandins can weaken tubal contractions, thus slowing down sperm transport and lessening the chances of them reaching the egg and fertilising it.

Another potential barrier for sperm is the large number of cells called macrophages found in the peritoneal fluid (bathing the abdominal organs) of women with endometriosis. Macrophages are scavenger white blood cells, and will quite happily gobble up sperm without realising their good intentions.

Immunology

Chapter 2 described how endometriosis could be an auto-immune disease in which the body starts to attack itself for some unknown reason. To summarise briefly, current theory suggests that the body's immune (defence) system recognises endometriosis as 'foreign' endometrium because it is not in its normal place lining the womb. The body then responds by producing antibodies against its own endometrium (these are called auto-antibodies). These may be merely incidental to the disease, or they may contribute to the inflammation associated with endometriosis, as antibodies help in the destruction of cells (though usually the cells that are destroyed are invaders of the body, such as bacteria). Anti-endometrium antibodies are in the blood of many women with endometriosis and, interestingly, their numbers only fall in women who respond well to drug treatment. Some evidence suggests that the chances of pregnancy only improve in women whose auto-antibody levels fall after treatment, implying that auto-antibodies may interfere with conception and/or implantation.

So, does mild endometriosis cause infertility?

As you can see, there is no easy answer to the question of whether mild endometriosis causes infertility. The evidence is often unhelpful because it is difficult to distinguish between cause and effect; for example, all the disturbances outlined above can occur both in women with severe disease and in infertile women who do not have endometriosis. These disturbances could just as easily be major causes of infertility in their own right, rather than ways in which endometriosis adversely affects fertility.

If finding endometriosis during the investigation of many women with infertility is a coincidence, then this would help explain why endometriosis is also found in women who have never had any trouble conceiving. And it would also suggest that the results of endometriosis research which relies on volunteers with infertility (who attend hospitals more often and tend to be willing subjects) may not apply to other women with endometriosis who conceive easily.

Perhaps the strongest evidence against mild endometriosis as a cause of infertility comes from studies where women were randomly allocated either treatment or a placebo (an inactive pill, see page 65), without knowing which one they were taking. There was no difference in the number of women who got pregnant in either group. Therefore, 'expectant management' or merely waiting for conception to occur naturally, with the reassurance that it will with time, is being increasingly recommended to infertile couples where the only problem is mild endometriosis.

On balance, the evidence suggests that endometriosis is a cause of infertility, but it is difficult to judge individual cases. This is partly because present methods for assessing how severe endometriosis is are not sophisticated enough (see Chapter 2) and much more needs to be understood about what seem to be definite defects in the way the ovaries and the immune system work in women with endometriosis.

TREATMENTS

Treatments for endometriosis designed to improve the chances of conceiving vary from hospital to hospital, as do the success rates. The treatment you are offered will obviously depend on how severe your endometriosis is and what you and your partner want, but it will also be influenced by your gynaecologist's experience of endometriosis and the facilities available.

The best hope of treating severe disease is to remove as much endometriosis and as many adhesions as possible and to restore the normal arrangement of your pelvic organs. As indicated in Chapter 4, this can be done during major surgery (laparotomy) or laparoscopic surgery. The advantages of the latter are a much shorter hospital stay and an easier recovery. Some doctors also claim that the risk of adhesions forming from the surgery itself is less. Unfortunately, laparoscopic surgery is not generally available in this country yet.

You may be advised to take drugs before or after surgery. Drug treatment before surgery may shrink some patches of endometriosis, reducing the amount of surgery necessary, and any areas not removed will be treated by drugs given after the operation. Unfortunately, endometriotic cysts rarely shrink and adhesions hardly ever disappear on drug treatment alone.

Mild endometriosis in women with infertility can be treated with either surgery or drugs, in much the way described in Chapters 3 and 4. Surgery is usually restricted to cauterising (burning away) the patches of endometriosis through the laparoscope. Although this has been a common practice for many years, its value has never been established. In some hospitals cauterisation may be done at the time of the first laparoscopy, and be the only treatment offered. One of a range of drugs may be suggested, with the recommendation that they are taken for six to nine months. Obviously, though, this has the disadvantage of delaying attempts to conceive until after treatment.

All the drugs available for treating endometriosis seem equally effective at improving infertility. Therefore what matters most is which one is easiest to take and has the least side effects, especially since you will be on it for quite a few months. You can be reassured that all current treatments have been shown to improve pregnancy rates, even if only slightly, in one study or another, although, having said that, research has also shown drug therapy and expectant management (otherwise known as positive thinking and keeping your fingers crossed) to be equally effective in mild endometriosis.

Summarising the success of the various treatments is an impossible task; claims for pregnancy rates following all these interventions range from 20–70 per cent, but studies are often not comparable because they are not done in the same way. Disease severity is often defined differently and the help of different sorts of patients is enlisted. Endometriosis may not be the only cause of the infertility being treated, and many studies only look at the problem with hindsight, which is a notoriously inaccurate way of conducting research.

FERTILITY DRUGS

Your doctor may suggest that you try fertility drugs, such as Clomid, to help you get pregnant. Clomid is best used to treat failure to ovulate; it is an anti-oestrogen drug, i.e. it lowers the levels of oestrogen circulating in the body. The pituitary gland responds to these very low oestrogen levels by producing more

FSH and LH, and sufferers often find their symptoms get worse temporarily as a result.

Several alternative medicines are said to improve fertility, including vitamin E, zinc and herbal extract vitex agnus castus (see Chapter 5). Approaches such as homoeopathy have also helped sufferers get pregnant.

IVF AND GIFT (ASSISTED CONCEPTION TECHNIQUES)

If treatment fails, or there is a coexisting problem such as your partner's poor sperm count, then you may be offered an assisted conception technique such as in vitro fertilisation (IVF) or gamete intra-Fallopian transfer (GIFT). In both cases, the idea is to stimulate the ovaries to produce a large number of eggs by giving daily injections of the gonadotrophins FSH and LH, contained in preparations such as Pergonal. Stimulation of the ovaries is monitored by measuring the diameters of the developing follicles with ultrasound, and when they have reached a certain maximum size an injection of human chorionic gonadotrophin (hCG) is given. This mimics the natural luteinising hormone (LH) surge in the menstrual cycle and helps the egg mature before ovulation. However, before ovulation can occur the eggs are gathered (harvested). At this stage the two techniques begin to differ.

With GIFT the eggs are harvested during laparoscopy under general anaesthetic. A needle is inserted into each follicle and the fluid, containing the egg, is aspirated (sucked up). The three best eggs, with sperm, are transferred into the end of the Fallopian tube via a fine tube. The aim is for fertilisation to occur naturally in the Fallopian tube.

With IVF the eggs are either harvested at laparoscopy, as described above, or using an ultrasound-directed technique that does not require a general anaesthetic. The easiest approach to the ovaries is via the vagina; an ultrasound probe placed there allows the ovaries to be 'seen' in great detail. A needle is then passed through the vaginal wall into the ovary to collect the eggs; most women are quite happy to undergo the procedure simply being sedated with Valium (to relax them) and pethidine (a painkiller). As many eggs as possible are then fertilised in the laboratory and, if embryos result, the

91

best three are inserted into the uterus two days after being collected. Some clinics freeze any embryos remaining after IVF so they can be thawed out and inserted in later menstrual cycles. Equally, any extra eggs obtained with GIFT can be fertilised in the laboratory and the resultant embryos frozen for later use.

Many IVF units are now suppressing the hormonal activity of the pituitary gland with LHRH analogues (see page 44) before stimulating the ovaries with Perganal. This yields more and better quality eggs, and also has the advantage of being a treatment for endometriosis at the same time.

Women with endometriosis tend to do well with IVF and GIFT but if they have extensive ovarian disease there is a tendency for fewer follicles to grow. There is a debate, though, about whether IVF or GIFT is better for women with endometriosis. The decision will partly depend on your partner's sperm, as there is a greater chance of fertilisation with IVF if the sperm are of poor quality. You must have at least one unblocked (patent) tube which is not stuck down with adhesions before you can have GIFT.

Success rates from the best clinics are very encouraging – 25–30 per cent of treatment cycles result in a pregnancy, using either technique. However, turned on their head, these figures indicate that the majority of couples entering treatment will not be successful. This uncertainty adds further stress to a very stressful form of treatment.

I have always had painful periods. However, three and a half years ago when we started trying for a baby, I found I had intermenstrual bleeding on and off during every cycle. My periods got heavier and heavier until that became more important to me than the gradual realisation that I might be infertile. One helpful doctor even suggested that it might be the excitement of a late marriage (age 27!) and the thought of a baby!!

To cut a very long story short, endometriosis was diagnosed by laparoscopy and I went into a nine-month-long nafarelin/danazol double blind trial (i.e. neither I nor my doctors knew what I was taking until after the research period). I was given Clomid almost as soon as I came off the trial. I had no side effects – only an almost overwhelming sense of hope at last. Indeed after four months on Clomid I did conceive, but sadly lost the 'pregnancy' two weeks later. We had been warned that the drug therapy would not cure the endometriosis and I might go back to square one and start intermenstrual bleeding again. I did not conceive again so we decided to try IVF.

The actual egg removal lasted an hour, there being 14 follicles. After four embryos were replaced, the waiting was rather stressful. We had been shown them on a video beforehand. I continually mentally monitored my body for any changes there might be. When the old familiar PMT symptoms came, it gradually dawned on me that it hadn't worked. It was worse for my husband. He thought of those embryos as 'babies' and he was sure it would work. I was not really optimistic but when you are desperate you are ready to try anything.

That was six months ago and we have recovered enough – financially and emotionally – to try again. We are going with less optimism this time, which I feel is the best way to approach IVF. It is easier to face the disappointment which, statistically, you are more likely to endure. If it doesn't work this time we will call it a day.

We are more at peace with ourselves now than we were after six months of 'trying'. It definitely starts to heal with time. Our friends have stopped trying to 'hide' new pregnancies which, in any case, never upset us. We have decided not to try and adopt – I think the process and the waiting would be much more traumatic than the IVF.

Endometriosis was diagnosed and danazol was prescribed for six months. After a second laparoscopy I was told I had three options: AID (artificial insemination with donor sperm), IVF and adoption. We decided to try IVF.

IVF is a very long process and tiring, but to reach fertilisation was good for us. But we were disappointed when a period started. Had we not applied to adopt I would most definitely have had a second attempt, despite the three week stay in London, and the Clomid and Pergonal injections, which were very painful.

As regards pregnancy, well I've almost accepted it may not happen – but we've been very lucky to adopt a little girl, Victoria, who was placed at seven weeks and is now two and a half. My infertility has been a great strain in my 14 years

93

of marriage, but after being determined and trying every way to have a baby, adopting Victoria has brought us much happiness. One tends to put the eight years of tests and IVF down to experience – you were pleased to have attempted but only too glad to forget.

My endometriosis was discovered about three years ago but my consultant believes I've had it for about eight years, as I've had pain all that time and heavy periods. I took danazol for six months and suffered from terrible side effects and still had endometriosis afterwards. I wasn't prepared to take it for another six months and, as a last resort, tried IVF. The pregnancy was a difficult one. Things have not been trouble-free since but we are grateful for having such a lovely child. It does seem an absolute miracle that she is here at all. We would love another baby and plan another attempt at IVF, but fully appreciate how fortunate we are in having one baby. Life is so much brighter now that Miriam is here.

Of course, just planning to try IVF or GIFT can sometimes do the trick.

I came off danazol after 18 months and went on to Clomid to try for another pregnancy (lost first at 11 weeks). The heavy bleeding and severe pain came back almost immediately and it was not long before it was continuous. I went back to my gynaecologist and asked for a hysterectomy, as this seemed the only way out. He said I had one more chance which was a procedure called GIFT. After discussing this with my husband, we decided to give it a go. When the time came for our appointment, to our amazement I had gone over three weeks with no bleeding and was beginning to wonder if I was pregnant. I was pregnant – to the surprise and delight of everyone.

UNDERSTANDING YOUR FEELINGS

Both endometriosis and infertility are long-term problems and each woman has to find her own way of coping. Women often feel a sense of failure and that they have let their partners and families down.

> Depression, frustration – I am a perfectionist. Guilt and sense of failure at inability to produce a baby.

> I find it hardest to handle the infertility and depression and 'feeling less than useless' syndrome that are part and parcel of it.

They also describe grieving over the loss of a potential child. Other people's expectations or insensitivity, or a friend's pregnancy, can bring back powerful feelings of broodiness just when you are feeling more confident.

Feelings of grief, anxiety and depression (see Chapter 8) are a natural response to the problems endometriosis and infertility can bring, and many women feel in need of support when they are trying to deal with them. Turning to your partner can be problematic since he will be going through his own jumbled feelings. Apart from his own sense of loss, he may be finding it difficult to support you in your upset, anger or depression. He may resent pain affecting your sex life, the need to 'perform' according to your charts or the general change in your life together. He may feel you aren't recognising his need for support. It is well known that infertility can strain relationships, but the added problems of endometriosis can make it even more difficult to stay in touch with each other.

> I had been hoping for another baby, but dreaded sex, which was often agonising, leaving me aching afterwards. This may have contributed to the breakdown of my marriage as my husband lost patience.

> The main problem for me has been the effect it has had on my marriage. What other disease could be so socially unacceptable – or should I say sexually unacceptable? The symptoms are enormously stacked against a smooth-running happy relationship – long heavy painful periods, painful intercourse, permanent exhaustion, mood swings, constipation and, worst of all, infertility. The constant surgery, both

minor and major, is extremely disruptive, and with the fear of total hysterectomy always just round the corner, it is very hard to relax and enjoy the everyday things in life which other women take for granted.

A husband writes a similar story.

My girlfriend became my wife in 1975 and about that time a consultant diagnosed 'endo-something or other'. She looked grotty for one week in every four, and often took to her bed with a hot water bottle and the painkillers. In 1976 the consultant said 'sorry, not much we can do, ever thought of a hysterectomy?' Our world fell apart. Constant problems. One week in four blacked out on the calendar – endless cancellations, silly excuses. Love-making a disaster; painful for her, and me full of fear of hurting her. In 1979 we knew we had a fertility problem – tests, trials, drugs and charts. In 1984 we couldn't take it any more – our marriage was almost on the rocks, we stopped going to the NHS infertility clinic and gave up hope of a family. However, we did go on a much-needed holiday and then decided to have one more try. A new approach, a new hope and as I write my wife is 12 weeks pregnant. For the first time in 10 years we look forward to the future together.

Turning to friends for support can also be difficult when most people don't know what endometriosis is and find infertility difficult to discuss. You may shy away from sharing your feelings after a few embarrassed silences or too much 'advice'. Attempts to protect you from their pregnancies can complicate old friendships.

A very close friend had an abortion and didn't feel able to tell me because of my endometriosis. I know she would have before.

Many women (and their partners) have found that it helps to share their feelings with others who have had similar experiences. This is possible through the Endometriosis Society or National Association for the Childless (NAC).

Since I had suffered from endometriosis for years before deciding to have children, my infertility should have come as no surprise: nevertheless, not becoming pregnant month after month soon became the hardest thing of all to accept.

A sympathetic doctor told me about NAC, but at the time I threw his leaflet into a drawer. No organisation with such a depressing name could be for me, and anyway I wasn't childless; just not pregnant yet! Several operations later and still no baby and I hit rock-bottom. We decided to join NAC and it was the best thing we ever did. At last we had a group of friends – infertile men as well as women – who understood and shared our problems. If you're one of the one in seven couples who are childless (or just not pregnant yet!) please join us.

FOSTERING AND ADOPTION

Adoption can be a happy solution to infertility.

My new life free of pain made the knowledge of my almost certain infertility easier to accept. Never for one moment did I feel cheated, hurt or depressed. My only concern was that my husband would feel unable to adopt. My fears were groundless. His thoughts were for providing for a child already brought into the world who was in need of parents. We adopted twin girls at the age of eight days and they have enriched our lives greatly. There have been moments when we are reminded that they are adopted, e.g. mums talking about confinements and people commenting on how one looks like 'Dad', the other like 'Mum', but we have taken these things in our stride. Adoption can be easy to forget – our daughters are simply our daughters.

In some cases adoption may not be that simple. Rules govern who is allowed to adopt (e.g. you will be ruled out if you are in your late 30s) and nowadays not as many babies need adopting. The adoption procedure can be long and complicated and raise new doubts about your ability to be a parent – which no one will have questioned during infertility investigations. It will also require a lot of commitment from your partner. By contrast, it is relatively easy to become a foster parent. This can be a very worthwhile experience, but some people find it difficult to make a short-term commitment when they were prepared to make a lifelong one, and others feel concerned about the amount of involvement social services want with fostered children. For further details write to British

Agencies for Fostering and Adopting (see useful addresses).

Becoming the parent of an adopted or fostered child can be an unexpected challenge when you don't have nine months' pregnancy to get used to the idea. You may also find it awkward being amongst other mothers (at last) and not being able to talk about pregnancy and childbirth. On the other hand, being able to share other pleasures and problems of having a young child will help you feel you belong. But be warned because adoption can have side effects!

I took Duphaston for 11 months, had another laparoscopy and was found to be clear. After that I took various fertility drugs which didn't work. However in June 1987 I found myself to be pregnant. I had a miscarriage and then a laparotomy which found a polycystic ovary and good old endometriosis. The endometriosis was removed and then I refused all other treatment for infertility. I just wanted to be left alone. In August we adopted seven-week-old Christopher. This was my best cure, I never felt better. However, in November we had a surprise – I found myself pregnant (no drugs or anything to help, only Christopher). Adopting Christopher was the best thing we ever did and because of him we are completing our family all in one year!

7

ENDOMETRIOSIS AND PREGNANCY

by Nicky Wesson

Once you are pregnant you are like other pregnant women, with all the same joys and sorrows. There are many books to help you (see recommended reading), but if you have endometriosis you may have some additional questions and find it difficult to get answers. This chapter looks at whether pregnancy can help reduce the symptoms of endometriosis, and whether having endometriosis can affect your pregnancy or your baby.

THE DECISION TO BECOME PREGNANT

If you are young, do not have children and have severe endometriosis, you may be told of the risk of infertility (see Chapter 6) and advised to become pregnant earlier rather than later. Pregnancy may also be recommended to you as a 'hormone treatment' for endometriosis. While it is true that pregnancy can reduce symptoms of the disease for some women, the idea that it will cure every sufferer for good is an out-of-date medical myth. An Australian study showed that 40 per cent of those who became pregnant had no further problems, but symptoms returned in the remaining 60 per cent, usually within one to four years of pregnancy (just when you would be dealing with an active pre-school child).

If you have a partner, want to have children together and are able to make the domestic and financial arrangements, you may be more than happy to have children sooner than you originally anticipated. On the other hand you may not be in this position, or you may feel that you do not want to be a mother and that changing your mind for the sake of 'treatment' is not good enough. Being confronted with the decision can be difficult.

I know they recommend pregnancy but it is just not possible at the moment. I do not feel ready to become a mother. But we are faced with a dilemma – do we wait until I am 30 and risk infertility or do we try soon when we do not really want to?

I was 22 and had just left university. It was hard to relate to what they said about the risk of infertility. I wasn't ready to settle down and my boyfriend didn't want kids. But when I saw a baby being born on TV, I burst into tears.

Although I want children, I feel to a certain extent I'm being pushed into it.

Even if your feelings about having children are fairly straightforward, they may be tinged with concern about your ability to conceive and carry the baby, and look after it if the endometriosis should return. If you do decide to get pregnant you can increase your chances of conceiving by making sure you (and your partner) are in good health. Good general advice is to stop smoking, gradually lose any extra weight, eat a healthy diet and reduce the amount of alcohol you drink. Various organisations provide further information about pre-conceptual care, e.g. Foresight (see useful addresses).

Some doctors suggest that you give your body a couple of months to get back to its normal menstrual cycle after drug treatment for endometriosis, before trying to conceive. This will not necessarily increase your chances of pregnancy, but at least your body will be back to normal before having to support a pregnancy. Sometimes ovulation can be delayed after hormone treatment, particularly with Primolut N and Provera, so you may want to take this into consideration when planning treatment in the hope of a subsequent pregnancy. Although endometriosis is associated with infertility in some women, many have got pregnant without any trouble, so do not be surprised if it works first time.

BEING PREGNANT

Little has been written about how endometriosis affects pregnancy, but some questions you may have might be answered by looking at two informal studies of sufferers who became pregnant. The first study, organised through the American Endometriosis Society, describes 187 out of 334 pregnancies in 187 women. A smaller British study collected information about 100 pregnancies in fifty-five women (a few of these occurred before the endometriosis had been diagnosed).

At first you may be surprised by your feelings when you discover you are pregnant, and in this respect sufferers are no different from other women. Many in the two studies described feelings of delight, but others had mixed feelings; even women who have been trying for a long time can feel confused when they eventually conceive:

Tired, bloated and scared stiff at the thought of having a baby (11 years trying to conceive).

If you have been pinning everything on pregnancy, the reality may fall short of your ideal image; you may feel trapped, or worry about things going wrong. These feelings are common amongst women, with or without endometriosis, so it may help to talk to friends who have been pregnant.

Does endometriosis mean you are more likely to have complications during pregnancy? Doctors sometimes assert that endometriosis sufferers are more likely to have a miscarriage, although there is no agreement about this in research papers. The rate of miscarriage amongst women in general is hard to assess since early miscarriage is not always reported or recorded, but it is generally put at 15–20 per cent of pregnancies confirmed by ultrasound or hearing the foetal heart. Including miscarriages before the foetal heart develops (which women often experience as a loss, even if the pregnancy was brief) would probably raise this figure considerably. When women in the two studies were asked if they had had a miscarriage, 34 per cent of the Americans and 30 per cent amongst the British said yes (the latter was increased by one woman who'd had ten miscarriages, although she managed to have four children). Some women report that homoeopathy and acupuncture have prevented miscarriage.

Bleeding during pregnancy can be a warning sign of a miscarriage, but 46 per cent of women in the British study had bleeding in the first four to five months which did not cause further problems. The bleeding ranged from spotting to heavy loss. This figure seems very high when compared to the 10 per cent for women in general in the first half of pregnancy. On the other hand, 16 reported bleeding without problems during the whole nine months in the American study. This suggests that bleeding during pregnancy may be more common amongst endometriosis sufferers, but need not be alarming. However, if you do suffer bleeding you should still check with your doctor at the time. Bed rest is often recommended, although there is no evidence that lack of rest is harmful.

You may experience unexpected pain during pregnancy – 54 per cent of the British women and 37 per cent of the American women complained of pelvic pain or cramping. Women in the British survey reported that pain often occurred in the early weeks, although some found it started later or lasted longer.

First three months very uncomfortable with lots of tummy pains due to adhesions being stretched.

Period-type aches in back and low abdomen and thigh aches for one to two months and at advanced pregnancy.

Considerable pain continues, sharp jagged pain all over.

All three pregnancies very uncomfortable and regularly quite painful. The first was the worst. I felt as though I was being stretched and torn inside my abdomen.

If stabbing pains are related to adhesions being stretched and separated by the changes in your uterus, they could even be beneficial! The surveys suggest that pain, often with bleeding, may be quite common without meaning anything is wrong – most women reporting these problems went on to have normal labours and healthy babies. However, to be sure you should contact your doctor. This is particularly important in the early months, as you may have an ectopic pregnancy (where the foetus starts to grow in the Fallopian tube, not the uterus) which is potentially very dangerous.

Of the British women, 33 per cent described the beneficial effects of pregnancy on their endometriosis pain.

Took several weeks for endometriosis pain to decrease, like

period pain – it was continuous but gone by eight to nine weeks.

Relief from endometriosis pain, PMT, mastitis [tender breasts], depression and irritability.

Total relief from endometriosis pain.

Wonderful relief, none of normal symptoms.

Of course, pregnancy also relieves premenstrual tension (PMT), which many sufferers report feeling during most of the month. This relief is probably temporary, as 59 per cent of those who suffered PMT before (67 per cent of British sample) found it was worse after the birth, 30 per cent felt there was no change and one or two felt it got better.

Far worse, two weeks before instead of a few days.

Yes, but much better, breasts not so painful, not so irritable, not so tearful.

Morning sickness is a less alarming problem which most women expect in the first three months of pregnancy, although studies estimate it only occurs in 30–50 per cent of pregnancies. However, 73 per cent of women in both the British and American studies reported nausea, which was often severe. In most cases, it had cleared by 14 weeks, although 12 British women suffered for most of the pregnancy. Nausea and vomiting were more common in first pregnancies. If this is a problem for you, alternative remedies can help and acupuncture before you conceive may prevent the problem (see recommended reading). GPs do not usually recommend drug treatment; if your GP does, discuss any worries you may have about its effects on the baby and check whether the drugs you are given will make you drowsy.

Extreme tiredness was often reported in the studies, but this is very common in all pregnant women (especially in the first three months) so it is impossible to judge whether this is worse for endometriosis sufferers. Evening primrose oil can help relieve fatigue during pregnancy.

You may wonder about taking nutritional supplements during pregnancy. This is a controversial issue, so you may prefer merely to pay attention to getting vitamins and minerals in your diet. None of the vitamin and mineral supplements described in Chapter 5 are known to cause damage during pregnancy. However vitamin A should not be taken in doses above 7,500 iu daily as this can cause malformation. Sufferers have recommended zinc for severe headaches during pregnancy.

CHILDBIRTH

There is no particular reason to think that your labour will be any different because you have endometriosis. In the British study the length of labour varied from 31 hours to 25 minutes, with an average of 11 hours, which is normal (taking into account that first labours are longer). Only three women had a caesarean section; two of these women felt the caesarean made their endometriosis symptoms worse, but a bigger study would be needed to find out if this was a common experience. A few cases of endometriosis in caesarean, amniocentesis or episiotomy scars have been documented in women who did not have a history of the disease previously.

Like women in general, women in the British survey often found labour very painful, but some felt it was easier to cope with than endometriosis pain.

Pain was bearable as, unlike endometriosis, you knew there was an end to it. I think that having endometriosis gives sufferers a much higher threshold of pain – I have found this in areas other than labour.

Women's experience of delivery varied, as one would expect, with 24 per cent having an induction, 18 per cent having forceps deliveries and 37 per cent having episiotomies. Some of these interventions were resented, particularly episiotomy. There are many books on childbirth (see recommended reading) to help you understand what you might be offered and decide what kind of birth you would prefer, given the opportunity. Talk to your doctors, your midwife, your partner and other women, and there are several organisations that can give you further information (see useful addresses). Antenatal classes teach breathing and pain-control techniques, which you may also find useful for endometriosis pain.

YOUR BABY

There is no reason to think that you will not have a healthy baby, but if you and your baby have problems you may worry that they are to do with your endometriosis or previous drug treatment.

Of the 60 babies recorded in the British survey, eight had some kind of abnormality. Most of these were minor and probably occurred at random. Fusion of the labia is the only condition that might be linked with drug treatment (see danazol in Chapter 3), although this has only been documented for women conceiving during treatment, not shortly afterwards. Surgical separation is possible.

Endometriosis does seem to run in some families (see Chapter 2), but long-term follow-up studies would be needed to find out how many daughters of endometriosis sufferers developed the disease. Current statistics suggest that your daughter probably will not get endometriosis, but if she does develop symptoms you can help her get prompt medical attention and make doctors aware of your history.

In the British study 55 per cent of the babies were described as having colic, where they cried painfully for long periods after feeding. This varied from a few days of mild colic to 'terrible' colic lasting for several months, well beyond the three months when colic is expected to end. There are no accepted guidelines about how common colic is, although one author comments that about 20 per cent of babies are generally expected to develop colic. The number of colicky babies in the British survey does seem comparatively high. Colic might be explained by a mother's *Candida albicans* infection (see Chapter 5) being passed on to the baby. If your baby is colicky or sleepless, there are books and organisations that give helpful advice (see recommended reading and useful addresses).

POSTNATAL DEPRESSION

It is normal to feel low a few days after having a baby, but 10–15 per cent of women also develop postnatal depression. This may develop gradually and can last months, even years. In the American study, 54 per cent felt depressed for eight

105

weeks, on average. This high rate may be related to the number of problems experienced during pregnancy. Postnatal depression can be particularly hard if you have already struggled with infertility.

> I made such a fuss about wanting a baby, but now I feel depressed and exhausted all the time and I'm so irritable, even with the baby.

The unanticipated exhaustion and emotional upheaval of caring for a baby can be very difficult, even when a child is dearly wanted. If you feel depressed, talk to your GP or try out alternative remedies such as cranial osteopathy, homoeopathy and acupuncture which have helped some women. It can help a lot to talk to other women and get outside support (see useful addresses).

BREASTFEEDING

The majority of babies in both studies were breastfed – 83 per cent of American and 82 per cent of British babies. British babies were breastfed for an average of eight to nine months but most lactating mothers found that their periods returned before this at about four to five months (compared to mothers who bottlefed, whose periods usually returned within two months).

Breastfeeding is recommended for many reasons, but some sufferers have also wondered whether it could delay their periods and their endometriosis returning. An Australian study reported that 60 per cent of 84 sufferers had a recurrence within 1–12 years of childbirth, and concluded that lactation did not necessarily delay endometriosis. However, in the absence of further research, it is worth a try. Most women in the American and British studies who did get a recurrence did not get symptoms before their first period.

If you want to lower your oestrogen levels and delay your periods by breastfeeding, you do need to follow a few guidelines. These will help ensure that your prolactin (milk-producing hormone) levels do not drop too much, allowing a return to your normal menstrual cycle.

- Breastfeed frequently (intervals of less than seven hours overnight, and at every meal).

- Breastfeed on demand, including through the night (or wake the baby for a feed before you go to bed).
- Do not give supplementary bottles. Express milk for a feed if someone else gives the bottle.
- Introduce solids late (six months or more).
- Consider breastfeeding into the second year, i.e. after 12 months.
- Try not to be embarrassed about feeding your baby in front of other people. If they get embarrassed, that's their problem!

CONCLUSIONS

The information about endometriosis and pregnancy is very limited and research with larger numbers of women would add to the informal American and British studies discussed in this chapter. There were wide variations in both studies, even within the experiences of pregnancy and babies in any one woman.

A few conclusions can be drawn though. If you have endometriosis, conceiving and maintaining a pregnancy is not necessarily going to be difficult, although it may well be uncomfortable, with a risk of bleeding, nausea and vomiting. The labour is not necessarily going to be longer or more difficult than usual. The baby may well cry more or sleep less than others and you could experience postnatal depression. However, all these problems have medical and alternative therapies. Vitamins and minerals may remedy some complaints. For those who get there, the outcome is felt to be well worthwhile – 'ecstatic', 'over the moon', 'worth it all'.

8

UNDERSTANDING YOUR FEELINGS

by Lesley Mabbett

On days free from pain and discomfort I feel great and can cope with any situation. When I don't feel well, even answering the telephone is traumatic.

I found that as the endometriosis progressed I had mood swings, lots of tearfulness, feelings of insecurity, anger and depression which I attributed to hormone imbalance or disturbance which I saw as very much part of the illness.

The emotional aspects of a chronic disease such as endometriosis can outweigh your physical symptoms. Sufferers often feel heightened emotions in response to being unwell, undergoing treatment and the disruption of daily life. Many people would argue that this is a natural reaction to any illness, but many endometriosis sufferers believe that their feelings could be a direct physiological result of their illness. Premenstrual syndrome, postnatal and menopausal depression have been ascribed to hormone changes which affect emotional states. Since women with endometriosis may also have hormone imbalances, and the drug treatments for endometriosis alter the hormonal control of the menstrual cycle, it is not surprising that sufferers often report feelings such as irritability, tiredness and depression.

This chapter looks at the many feelings women with endometriosis can have and their need for emotional support as well as treatment of the disease. If you suffer from endometriosis, you will probably discover that you are not alone in some of your hopes and fears, and many women have found that sharing their feelings is a big step towards feeling better.

FEARS AND ANXIETIES

Fears and anxieties are probably the first feelings you can remember about your endometriosis. They naturally accompany the distressing symptoms and your not knowing what is wrong.

I have always found not knowing the cause of the pain almost more difficult to bear than the pain itself.

The worst thing about the whole time was the loneliness, the fear that I could actually cause such pains by neurosis and the final terror (subconscious at first) that I might have cancer.

Having a name for what you've got is often an enormous relief because it puts these fears to rest.

I was so glad to realise I probably had a complaint with a name; it was something to go and investigate for myself.

Diagnosis is only the beginning, though. Endometriosis sufferers soon find there are other things to worry about.

I am finding it all very frightening – the hormone treatment and its effects, the possibility of hysterectomy and, of course, the threat of infertility.

Fears and anxieties often arise from lack of information. Although information can give you more to worry about, in general people are more anxious about the unknown and what they don't understand. So finding out about endometriosis and its treatment may allay some of your concerns and help you assess your situation more realistically. Talking to people can help you to put things in perspective – realising that other sufferers share your anxieties may help you accept that these concerns are a natural part of coping with endometriosis.

Some people are more prone to anxiety than others, and research in Belgium suggests that endometriosis sufferers may be amongst them. Talking to your doctor or gynaecologist (see Chapter 2) can help you take your anxieties into account when reaching decisions about treatment. For example, will you be better off having your ovaries removed if you are terrified of losing your femininity and sexual relationship, even if this does wonders for your endometriosis? Your fears need to be recognised and discussed before you reach a decision.

If anxiety starts taking over your life (e.g. with panic attacks), or crippling fear is preventing you from going for the surgery you need, your GP may be able to refer you to a clinical psychologist.

GRIEVING

When you learn you have endometriosis, you may grieve for lost hopes and expectations. It isn't easy to come to terms with the fact that endometriosis prevents you from doing some of the things that you want to do in life, or being the person that you want to be, such as becoming a mother or being someone who isn't ill, being a lover who isn't worried about pain on intercourse, or someone who has more energy for their job, family, friends and hobbies. Grieving is expressing your feelings about such lost opportunities.

Psychologists studying loss and ways of helping the bereaved have noticed that people often go through stages of grieving. Your feelings may not match these stages exactly, because endometriosis sufferers go through periods of hope and doubt (especially if they have to try a variety of treatments) rather than a single loss as in divorce or the death of a loved one.

Denial
I was unable to accept this had happened.

Imagine a situation in which you really feel like crying but are holding back the tears. All your attention is focused on not crying, so it is hard to concentrate on anything else. Are there any tears that you are holding back about endometriosis? What about your other feelings? You may have buried your feelings about the pain or infertility, to stop them overwhelming you and the other people that care about you.

Although this is a very common way of coping, it takes a huge amount of nervous energy to act as if 'everything's OK'. You may feel perpetually exhausted and unable to direct your energies to dealing with the disease.

In some ways acting as if you haven't got a pain when you have is quite a lonely and estranging experience. My

111

husband insists that I am honest with him about how I really am, and that helps a geat deal.

By all means have a good cry, it can be very therapeutic.

When I read the leaflet about endometriosis, I just sat and cried for ages. The grief was for all the years spent feeling that pain (particularly pain during and after sex, or being doubled up in agony on the bedroom floor during a period) was an inevitable part of being a woman and that to complain was wimpish, childish and probably a form of attention-seeking.

Denial of an illness can also take the form of unrealistic expectations. Often this is not helped by your doctor's reluctance to admit the limitations of current treatments (see Chapters 3 and 4) or the possibility of endometriosis returning before your menopause. Even if this has been explained, the natural tendency is to assume that your treatment will cure you and not to think until later about what you're going to do if it doesn't. Women have described how they felt unable to get on with their lives because they were waiting – to get better or to conceive, for example. Life improved when they reassessed their expectations and began to make decisions for the here and now, even if this meant accepting their limitations and finding new ways to manage.

After several years of no social life, I hope to establish some nights out and see how I can cope with a normal life.

During these months my husband and I came to terms with the fact that we would probably never have children, and rearranged our lives accordingly.

Ironically, a perpetual search for the magic answer may get in the way of real healing. The classic example is when women find that accepting their infertility and making new plans suddenly does the trick.

My partner and I discussed yet another op, but decided against it – we started to plan our lives ahead without the patter of dainty feet. I decided that this 'thing' in my body, endometriosis, was going to stop ruling my life and I began to take control, relaxing more, learning to breathe and doing lots more exercise walking the dog than I'd ever done in my life. I began to feel alive again – and got pregnant! It was a shock to us both, and initially not really wanted. We'd mapped out a new life which didn't include a baby! But now our baby is wanted so much, I can't wait until July when it is due.

Withdrawal and isolation
Lacking in confidence, irrational insecurity and feelings of complete isolation at times.

Endometriosis often causes women problems which make them feel isolated or want to withdraw from people. Gynaecological complaints are not exactly an easy topic of conversation and most people have never heard of endometriosis. Your attempts to explain it may make you wish you hadn't bothered.

I thought that there was only me that suffered from this as no one had ever heard of it before. When they ask me what's wrong when I don't feel well and I try to explain, they look at me as though I'm silly. No one really knows what we go through.

People often react to someone who develops a chronic illness as they do when someone is bereaved. After initial sympathy and offers of help, they find it difficult to cope with their feelings and don't like to think of it going on and on. Lack of understanding gives them unrealistic expectations.

The trouble is, being treated in hospital, my boss and everyone else presumes I'm cured and so it is difficult explaining that it's always there.

Your response may be to withdraw from friendships and a social life. Endometriosis can also make you feel isolated in close relationships.

Endometriosis puts a severe strain on myself personally and my partner. This is due to changes of mood, lack of sex drive, tiredness and the constant threat of things being spoilt by pain. I feel that since the illness I have become much more withdrawn.

It is only natural to feel sorry for yourself at times, but if you find you are 'enjoying' sitting alone listening to sad music or dwelling on things that have happened to you (yes, other

113

people have done it too!), then it's time to find support (see page 124 and the list of useful addresses).

Anger

Endometriosis can give you plenty to be angry about. You may feel it has ruined your sex life, made your job a struggle or impossible, prevented you from having children or made coping with relationships difficult. Your symptoms may have dragged on in spite of your remembering to take tablets for nine months or having major surgery. Anger about your life is quite understandable.

> Even if it happens to other women, it still affects *my* life, creating tension and unhappiness in my marriage.

You have every reason to be angry about this suffering, yet many women find anger a particularly hard emotion to express. They go through cycles of feeling extremely irritable and then guilty because they have taken it out on other people.

> My biggest regret as a result of this disease is the way I have treated my children. I shout very loudly when I should be calmly explaining what they are doing.

> Family fed up with mother's moans, husband living like a monk, tempers and tears, etc.

Paradoxically, it makes sense to take your feelings out on those you love, because they are least likely to reject you for doing it, but cracks may begin to show in relationships if this carries on for too long.

> The constant pain for months made me irritable. My marriage was threatened for a while as my husband was unable to understand why I was a permanent 'cross patch'.

Your partner may also feel frustrated by the disease continuing and your perpetual need for support, which may not be forthcoming after a while, unless you give yourselves a chance.

> We both like walking, and this can be a very good way of relaxing and leaving your troubles behind. It also gives you a chance to talk.

If you seek outside help (see pages 124-6) invite your husband or partner to get support for his difficulties living with the disease too.

Unexpressed anger can turn into self-destructive feelings of depression.

> Felt diagnosis was very slow and spent a long time convincing male doctors that I had a gynaecological problem (after first laparoscopy showed nothing). Was given all kinds of irrelevant tests and felt very low about this.

No, it isn't easy to get angry with doctors (see Chapter 2), but if you are clear and assertive at least you know that you've done what you can to improve communication. If you feel that a doctor didn't diagnose endometriosis or warn you of side effects during drug treatment, then try writing a letter. Perhaps you won't send it, but writing it all down will help. And who knows, if you do write and tell doctors the final diagnosis or the benefits of knowing what side effects to expect, it could help their future patients.

If you feel like shouting at God or fate for letting you get endometriosis, then let your feelings out – God is perhaps the only one big enough to take everything you can throw at Him without giving up on you. Or you can scrub the floor vigorously or knead bread instead. Or try this bioenergetics exercise, perhaps with someone safe around to support and encourage you: make a big pile of cushions and kneel in front of it. Take a deep breath in as you raise your fists over your head and then shout as you bring your fists down on the cushions. Repeat until you feel better.

Endometriosis can give you enough feelings of anger to deal with without taking in any more. So if bureaucrats, shopworkers or queue-jumpers annoy you, let them know as calmly as possible. Similarly, try to confront friends and colleagues as constructively as possible with grievances against them. Assertiveness techniques can help a great deal (see recommended reading).

Guilt and blaming

No one knows what causes endometriosis. If you have heard people use expressions like 'career woman's disease', you may blame yourself for not having had children earlier, without realising that this term is based on the unproven idea that women who delay childbearing are more susceptible to endometriosis. Or you may feel it is your fault you did not get an earlier diagnosis.

I deeply regret not being more assertive when possibly an earlier diagnosis could have been made. I just accepted that I was over-sensitive to pain. I was my own worst enemy.

It is easy to get into a vicious circle, where you feel a victim and blame yourself for causing or contributing to the disease and then feel guilty about the feelings.

At the beginning of my illness I became very depressed, insular and moody. This generates a feeling of constant worry and guilt because it sorely affects what I, or my partner and I, can do.

'Don't blame yourself' is easier said than done, but it can help if you assume responsibility only for things you can actually change now. Maybe you shouldn't have used the coil. Were you under too much stress, or eating the wrong foods? Until more is known about endometriosis, you won't know the answers, and perhaps not even then.

And say you found out using the coil was a cause. Blaming yourself after the event will not help. Being more assertive might have led to an earlier diagnosis (you don't know), but you did what you could at the time and it is difficult to judge how serious symptoms are and how much to push your doctor.

Depression
Everything is just too much trouble.

There have been times recently when I wished myself in heaven.

Depression seems to be very common amongst endometriosis sufferers. In the Endometriosis Society survey, 63 per cent said that depression was a symptom of their endometriosis (see page 14). Comments suggested that many respondents felt depressed because problems seemed out of their control.

I think I become depressed because I experience a lot of pain and see no hope of a cure. Also I am depressed by my inability to have a normal sex life.

Feeling very helpless because of lack of treatment and disinterest of doctors. Every day is the same, with no relief from pain and no pleasure because of pain and tiredness.

116

Equally, others have described how much regaining control helped their feelings and physical symptoms, through finding out more, meeting others, making decisions positively, trying alternative approaches, or adopting a new lifestyle (see Chapters 5 and 9). Remember you are just as likely as anyone else to suffer from premenstrual syndrome, postnatal depression, weepiness after surgery, menopausal depression (see recommended reading and useful addresses for help) and the commonplace ups and downs of everyday life.

Depression in fact can range from a relatively mild feeling of being 'down' to a condition which affects every aspect of life and becomes a threat to your well-being.

I am completely unable to enjoy life in any way. I neither laugh nor cry, I have no feelings at all – I feel like a robot. I am worried and forgetful and sometimes my mind literally goes blank.

If you have feelings like these, lack of appetite and early waking, you could well be suffering from clinical depression. You may also find that you start to use (or use more) alcohol, sleeping pills, tranquillisers or other drugs to help you cope.

If the depression gets to a point where it is having a damaging effect on your work, your family or your life in general, or if you are having suicidal thoughts, do go and see your GP before things get any worse. A short course of anti-depressant drugs may relieve the situation. It may also be possible to get counselling or psychotherapy on the NHS (see page 125).

Acceptance and resolution

Acceptance is the final stage of grieving. No one would suggest that acceptance after bereavement means that you forget the loved one or stop caring that he or she died. Similarly coming to terms with endometriosis is slowly accepting that you have the disease, that it may or may not get better or worse, that it limits you in several ways, but that it is not the whole of life and there are still many joys and achievements open to you, including some you have not yet considered (e.g. making new friends through a self-help group). When you come to terms with endometriosis you begin to feel better physically and emotionally.

For me the worst thing was not being able to have a baby. This has been the biggest disappointment in my life, causing tremendous distress throughout the years. However, this is now behind me and I have learnt to come to terms with this situation, although there are times when I feel a bit down.

I think we can only get better at the point where we stop asking 'them' to cure us and take responsibility for ourselves. That's quite a burden and in my case it was autogenic training (see page 142) that helped me take it on. I've still got endometriosis, but I'm not being destroyed by it.

If the idea of acceptance seems utterly impossible to you, you are probably still battling through other feelings. Coping with endometriosis is not an easy matter, nor is it a once-and-for-all thing. A recurrence of pain, or a sister or friend having a baby, can cause setbacks, upsetting the equilibrium you had reached.

CHICKEN OR EGG?

I sometimes feel I reacted emotionally to situations in my life because I felt so unwell. On the other hand it could be that emotional stress worsened, aggravated and possibly caused the endometriosis.

Researchers in Belgium, the United States and Britain are now becoming interested in the connection between endometriosis and emotional states and the possibility that stress contributes to its development. Sufferers often describe problems in childhood or traumatic life events before their endometriosis began.

My first husband left me in May 1975. Up to that time my periods were absolutely normal and like clockwork. From that date I went through a traumatic period. I met my second husband in August 1975, we married in 1977 and it was approximately six months later that the symptoms began.

Of course, everyone goes through a lot of problems so it may just be that there is always something you can pinpoint before your endometriosis started. However, research suggests that stress can upset the unconscious parts of the brain which control the hormone (endocrine) and defence (immune) systems. There is increasing evidence that disorder in the immune system allows endometriosis to develop and that imbalanced hormones assist its growth (see Chapter 2).

It is too early to conclude from research that emotional states contribute to or cause endometriosis, but the experience of sufferers does suggest that dealing with emotional problems and other stresses can reduce physical symptoms of the disease and encourage positive feelings.

HELPING YOURSELF

Find out as much as possible

I feel I could face up to the condition better if I had more information about the outcome of different options.

The relief at finding an explanation was enormous.

Most sufferers want to know more about endometriosis and its treatment. Reading this book is a good start! Plenty of information exists on related issues, such as infertility, having a hysterectomy, going through the menopause or alternative treatments (see recommended reading and useful addresses). The Endometriosis Society newsletter provides current information and describes what other sufferers have found helpful.

However all the information can be a bit confusing. You will not find straightforward answers; for example, you may have noticed that this book talks about 'pros and cons' of treatments and 'chances' of success. Without proper research, statements of fact by doctors and alternative practitioners may in reality merely be a matter of opinion. There is nothing wrong with opinions as such – after all, practitioners are trying to help women with endometriosis and what they are suggesting may well be worth trying – but it does mean you will come across conflicting views about the best approach. If you investigate all the alternatives you will feel happier about the final decision.

Making decisions

Having endometriosis involves one decision after another, although at some stages you may not be given any options.

You may find decision-making is straightforward, or you may feel angry and rushed without the necessary information or time to think about it.

The specialist recognised endometriosis and recommended I have a hysterectomy, which I decided to have.

The amount of time a patient gets in the NHS outpatients is totally inadequate for the patient. The communication was terse, information limited, information exchange inadequate. Yet these are big decisions that need talking over.

Most people's decision-making is based on a mixture of thoughts and feelings. The best option is usually clear in simple decisions, and being wrong may not matter, but sufferers of endometriosis are often faced with complicated choices, for example about treatment or becoming pregnant.

Being more systematic in making difficult decisions can help you feel more confident and avoid later surprises or regrets. The accompanying box gives an outline of one way you may approach a decision. Although it looks very logical it does not exclude feelings you may have – these may seem irrational, but are none the less important.

QUICK GUIDE TO MAKING DECISIONS

- What is the problem?
- Is it important enough to spend time thinking about it?
- If yes, seek more information and help, e.g. from doctors, family and friends, support group, for the next steps.
- What are your alternatives?
  What is likely to happen in each case?
  What are the immediate advantages and disadvantages?
  What are the long-term advantages and disadvantages?
  How do you feel about each alternative and any risks you might have to take?
- Can you try any of them out and change your mind?
  Are you prepared to accept the consequences of those you cannot reverse?

If you are faced with an important decision, it will help to explore your options – and remember that doing nothing and waiting to see what happens is also one of these options. This chapter suggests many ways of getting further information and discussing the problem with women who have had similar experiences. Your decision may involve other people – your partner for example – and you will need to get their reactions. Do you know what their feelings are? Are you making any assumptions about them?

Once you have worked out your options assess the chances of success in each case, e.g. chances of conception with IVF, (page 92), chances of recurrence if ovaries remain (page 53). Then think of the advantages and disadvantages in the immediate and long-term. For example, danazol is likely to stop the pain but you may get side effects (at which point you could try evening primrose oil to combat them, or stop taking danazol). Danazol may help you get pregnant in the longer term but it is not the answer if you have cysts. Surgery is a better alternative for cysts but it is unpleasant initially and you will need time to recuperate. Or think about an alternative approach; surgery could stop pain and make you feel more positive, but you may need to find a good practitioner and be able to pay.

You will obviously have feelings about each choice, but sometimes the real reasons you do or don't like a particular option can be difficult to pinpoint. You may think it is silly to feel a particular way.

When I had both ovaries removed I thought I would age very quickly.

You shouldn't look upon these emotions as silly, though. 'Silly' feelings are real and part of examining all the options. Your commitment to a sensible decision may be sapped, under-mined, by the silly feelings underneath – they are therefore not silly, but important, and have to be faced up to and sorted out. It may require a bit of careful thought and honesty with yourself, but if you let the feelings out then you can check your worries. You need to take into account your personal hopes and fears. If you dearly wish to conceive, you will probably opt for the treatment most likely to help, even if it may require a lot of effort. If you want to control pain, your choice may be different. Other priorities may be to maintain a good relationship with your partner, to feel good about yourself, to carry on with work or to avoid taking drugs all the time. You may have short-term goals as well, such as being fit to go on the holiday of a lifetime, not having surgery during exams, feeling fit for an interview, etc.

Your priorities may not be the same as your doctor's, so it is worth discussing with him or her what you want any treatment to achieve. Your doctor may put your physical health before other things which you see as equally important, e.g. feeling sexually attractive, the need to take account of domestic arrangements. Talking to your doctor is a chance for concerns to be expressed before the final decision. This advice may seem rather irrelevant if your doctor is not actually offering you a choice. However, it is your health at stake, so you can ask for time to consider the matter and you do have the power to say no. You may be afraid of offending the doctor, but to do so is better than the shock of discovering you have not understood what is being suggested and of feeling the decision has been made for you.

> She recommended hysterectomy and finally sterilised me, without proper counselling and advice, and caused me great grief and sorrow when I realised I could not have another child.

Getting in touch with others
My family and friends have been very helpful and supportive since my endometriosis was diagnosed but there has still been that isolated feeling of 'no one understands'. Now I know that lots of women understand – only too well!

I felt so elated because at last I could mention endometriosis and the whole group 'tuned in' and gave their experiences. We had a really good group therapy session. The leaflet read like a diary of my thoughts, feelings and fears.

Self help groups give you the opportunity to share your feelings with other people who know what it is like to have endometriosis. They can help you feel less isolated, and you may also feel better about talking to your doctor ('I didn't know anything about endometriosis so I didn't even know what questions to ask'). Some self-help groups teach new skills, such as pelvic-floor exercises and relaxation techniques, or simply provide a social night out and a way of making new friends.

Certain sessions may be open to partners and husbands, giving them a chance to learn about endometriosis and to share their feelings.

Participating in or running a group can do wonders for feelings of helplessness and anger. It allows women to feel that at last they have found a way of fighting the disease by helping themselves and others.

The Endometriosis Society produces regular newsletters and provides a telephone/penpal scheme and a network of self-help groups throughout the UK. The National Association for the Childless and the Hysterectomy Support Group are amongst other organisations who provide newsletters and run local support groups (see useful addresses).

Religious faith

Surveys in Britain indicate that the majority of people believe in God, although only about 15 per cent are regular worshippers. You may see religion as a positive or negative force when coping with endometriosis. Many people's early religious upbringing will have included a good deal of moral teaching, especially about the role of women; for example, some religious cultures regard infertility as a sign of God's displeasure. This kind of teaching may contribute to a feeling that you are being punished for something; many sufferers ask 'What have I done to deserve this?' inferring that they are being held to blame.

All religions have to deal with the problem of why 'good' or 'innocent' people suffer. In the Jewish and Christian traditions the problem is tackled in the Bible in the Book of Job. The easy solution is to maintain, as Job's friends did, that the sufferer must be to blame in some way, but the conclusion of the book is more difficult to comprehend. God is portrayed as both loving and all-powerful and that, while He has each individual's best interests at heart, they may not be able to understand how His love and power are manifested.

As an aside, it is worth noting that the Bible is full of women who were infertile for years. Although their culture would have held them to blame, their histories show them as essential figures whose anguish made it possible for the birth of a child to be a special event and a turning point in the Biblical story. Jesus had only praise for the woman with a menstrual disorder who dared to touch Him for his healing.

123

Charismatic religious movements place great emphasis on faith and prayer for healing. However, it doesn't always work, and the sufferer may then feel terribly guilty and that she is to blame.

A friend who is also a Christian wanted to pray for me and lay hands on me to heal. I must admit I was a bit reluctant at first and thought it was a little bit funny, but I went. Nothing happened. I still had pain. I know now it was because I had no faith.

Faith itself is described as 'not of ourselves, it is the gift of God'. Some women have found greater peace through seeing God as someone who wants to love rather than to blame them.

With some close friends we started to pray for a complete healing. Rather than shaking my fist at God because he wouldn't give me a child, I began to realise his plans went deeper. The complete peace of mind that Jesus talked about came when I listened to God as a wise father and gave up expecting him to justify Himself by doing as I demanded. I learned to accept myself as complete without a baby and to stop comparing myself with other women. Exactly a year ago today a pregnancy was confirmed.

Other sources of support

People often tell horror stories about their doctors. (Your doctor probably feels the same way about builders or plumbers!) However many women have found their GP, gynaecologist or nurses very supportive. This is not to excuse those in medicine or nursing who have caused a lot of unnecessary grief or misunderstanding, but any profession is a mixture of people, and support and understanding will be available from somewhere.

Nursing staff were very kind and held my hand while I cried it all out of my system.

My husband and I would have given up more than once, but my gynaecologist does not give up easily and we are grateful to him for getting us this far.

It was fully explained to me by my own GP, who has been a tower of strength throughout the entire time.

Someone, somewhere understands and cares. Don't give up until you've exhausted every possibility that is available to you.

If you are unhappy with your GP or gynaecologist, then you can go elsewhere (see page 28). However it may be that a doctor – any doctor – is simply not in a position to provide the emotional support you need, in which case you may need to become a member of a self-help group instead or consider other possibilities such as counselling, co-counselling or group therapy. They may sound a bit trendy, but sufferers have found them helpful.

A good counsellor can help you explore your emotions, your relationships with others and your feelings about treatments or decisions you have to make, rather than tell you what to do. A psychotherapist can help you think at a deeper level by looking at damaging experiences in early life and ways in which you have adopted negative emotional or behavioural patterns to cope, which may no longer be helpful now and may be contributing to your problems or to the endometriosis itself.

Counselling or therapy helps you change in positive ways. You may be afraid of exposing feelings you would rather not admit even to yourself. No one will force you to talk about them, but people often find a weight lifts when they reach a stage where they feel able to. You may also feel that going to someone for psychological help for endometriosis means admitting 'that it's all in your head'. You are certainly not declaring yourself mentally ill by seeking help: instead you are recognising that endometriosis is causing emotional problems which you can't resolve on your own and that going for help is a way of restoring your well-being.

Your GP or consultant may be able to refer you locally, although counselling and psychotherapy are limited on the NHS. Several voluntary organisations offer counselling services, but you will need to find out what is available in your area. Try contacting the British Association for Counselling or your local branch of MIND (the Mental Health Association) or the Samaritans for advice about local services or lists of counsellors. The Westminster Pastoral Association will put you in touch with a counsellor who can take account of your spiritual needs, if you wish. Relate (formerly known as the Marriage Guidance Council) or the Child Guidance Service provide help where problems have become focused on an area of family relationships (look them up in the phone book). Women's Therapy Centres are another possible source of help. You will often have to see a counsellor privately, which can be expensive – £15–£25 an hour is not uncommon – but some organisations operate a sliding scale of charges, so it is worth asking before you decide you can't afford it.

Co-counselling is a technique in which you are paired with someone and take it in turns to focus on the other's problems, meeting on a regular basis and sticking to certain guidelines. It has the advantage of being cheap and flexible, but you may find you need the skills and insight of a trained counsellor, or that you feel too needy to be able to offer much to someone else.

As for group therapy, there are innumerable varieties. You can find out what might suit you from *A Complete Guide to Therapy* (see recommended reading). The organisations mentioned above and women's health centres may know of suitable groups in your area.

I have found group therapy very effective in helping with emotional aspects of being ill and in redirecting energies wasted in worrying.

9

GETTING TO GRIPS WITH PAIN

by Lesley Mabbett

For most sufferers, endometriosis *is* pain. You know you've got the disease or that it has returned because you recognise the pain. Many women might not mind being riddled with endometriosis if it didn't affect fertility and cause pain. Some doctors have gone so far as to suggest that, since treatment for endometriosis is long, often with unpleasant side effects, and surgery can result in scarring, they should treat the pain rather than the endometriosis (unless pregnancy is desired).

This chapter dwells on pain in order to illustrate the ways in which endometriosis sufferers have tried to change their lives, deal with their pain and look towards a brighter future.

> Since stopping the tablets I still feel very well. It might be because I am free of monthly pain for the first time in my life and that does the trick. It is an indescribable feeling.

> I feel better now than I have done for 20 years and it is so good to be able to plan things ahead.

ENDOMETRIOSIS AND PAIN

Women with endometriosis report many types of pain, but ironically endometriosis is not necessarily painful. Sufferers can have severe endometriosis and no painful symptoms (see Chapter 2). Pain probably arises because of where the endometriosis is and the inflammation and scarring it causes.

Endometriosis can irritate and inflame the peritoneum (the membrane lining the abdominal cavity), which produces prostaglandins (found in unusually high levels in some

94% suffer from
period pain,
severe for 66%.

Cramps extend down my legs to my knees and sometimes to my ankles I am in extreme pain from my waist to my toes.

77% have ovulation
pain, severe for 30%.

A DULL ACHING NAGGING PAIN ON RIGHT SIDE AT OVULATION, GOING DOWN INTO MY VAGINA

57% experience
pain at any time
of the month.

A definite bruising feeling from one hip bone to the other. On the days without pain the whole area feels as if I had been kicked.

55% have painful
sexual intercourse.
3% said this meant
they couldn't try for
a baby.

Sharp pain on deep penetration. Much worse in certain positions.

48% suffer painful
defaecation.

6-7 days before onset of periods pain on opening bowels

37% get back pain
during periods.
42% have it most
of the time.

BACK-PAIN, SOMETIMES DURING PERIODS OR AT OVULATION, WITH PAIN IN THE RIGHT LEG

32% are kept
awake by apin.

I found I could not sleep on my back or sides so I used to "sit-up" with the aid of many pillows

26% found urination
caused pain.

SEVERE PAINS IN THE FRONT PASSAGE PAINFUL TO START URINATION & MAINTAIN A FLOW OF URINE

Common pains reported by sufferers in the Endometriosis Society
Survey.

sufferers). Prostaglandins are hormone-like chemicals produced by the body which, among other things, can stimulate
pain nerve endings or cause spasmodic contractions in the
uterus which feel like intense 'period' pains and backache. An
acute attack of severe pain on the left or right side of the pelvis
can mean a chocolate cyst on one or other ovary has ruptured,
causing intense irritation of the peritoneum.

Adhesions can cause pain after the endometriosis has gone
because internal organs are stuck together in uncomfortable
positions. This may account for dragging sensations, painful
bowel movements, painful sex and sharp pains in pregnancy or
due to sudden movement when adhesions are pulled.

Some researchers have suggested that unexplained pelvic
pain (in women in general) may be due to congestion of veins
flowing through the pelvis, and this may also apply to
endometriosis sufferers who can have extra fluid in the pelvic
cavity.

However, doctors do not really know how endometriosis
causes pain, or why the pain is so severe in some sufferers, yet
doesn't appear in others. The fact that it is difficult to measure
hampers research and can make it hard to convince your
doctor about the extent of your pain, especially when it isn't
related to the amount of endometriosis.

The surgeon's visual inspection indicates that it's not severe.
However, I find the pain crippling, and totally inhibiting to
my usual lifestyle.

My GP was helpful but both he and the consultant took a
long time to take account of the terrible pain it caused.

If a pain meter could give an instant reading, perhaps your
doctor would be more helpful. Try using the pain chart
overleaf to record your pain. Although it will be subjective, it
may help your doctor understand what you are going through.
Or use it to see how well some of the pain-relief methods
described in this chapter work for you.

HOW PAIN RELIEF WORKS

Put simply, pain is a message from a part of your body which
is suffering damage or going wrong, telling your brain to do

Pain scale.

something about it. Pain relief interrupts the transmission of the pain message at different points along its path. Research suggests that dull aches travel by one route into the brain, while sharp stabbing pains pass along another – which explains why some pain-relief methods affect one type of sensation while leaving the other untouched.

Aspirin and related drugs block the production of prostaglandins, reducing any inflammation and interfering with the formation of pain messages at nerve endings. Narcotic drugs block pain messages at critical sites in the spinal cord and brain. One way they do this is by imitating endorphins, chemicals which are the body's natural painkillers. Both narcotics and endorphins can attach to receptors in the brain and spinal cord producing a painkilling effect and a feeling of well-being. Endorphins can be stimulated by sustained exercise

130

such as running and aerobics, and by using techniques such as acupuncture and shiatsu to treat pain.

The way pain is perceived once it reaches the brain depends on attitudes, expectations, thoughts and feelings. For example, research suggests that distracting people can reduce their pain by as much as a third. On the other hand, if you're expecting to hurt, or perhaps if the suffering actually rescues you from an unpleasant situation, you may be unconsciously concentrating on the pain. The mechanism for this is not well understood.

THE MEDICINE CABINET

Over-the-counter medicines

Several mild painkillers are available at the pharmacist. Aspirin reduces any fever and inflammation, as well as killing pain, but it can cause stomach irritation and bleeding. These side effects can be reduced by taking it with food or milk, using soluble tablets, or trying another drug in the salicylate family (e.g. benorylate, salicylamide although you may need a prescription for this). Ibuprofen is another popular anti-inflammatory and mild painkiller, but it can also irritate the stomach lining. Paracetamol is a good alternative painkiller if you cannot tolerate these side effects, but it does not reduce inflammation.

You will find many brands of aspirin or paracetamol or both. There is no evidence that combinations of these drugs are more effective and it is often an expensive way of taking them. You may be surprised to find caffeine included in some preparations. It may make the painkiller more effective, but it is a stimulant and can keep you awake at night. Read the label to make sure what any compound contains – and don't take even mild painkillers for more than ten consecutive days without medical advice. Do discuss over-the-counter drugs with your GP because they can interact with other medicines.

Anti-spasmodic drugs in the hyoscine family can relieve period pain. Endometriosis sufferers have found Feminax, which includes this type of drug, a useful standby so it is worth a try if you can tolerate all its ingredients (salicylamide, paracetamol, codeine, hyoscine hydrobromide and caffeine). Read the label for precautions, because anti-spasmodics can cause nausea and drowsiness.

If you want a stronger painkiller, you can buy many preparations containing codeine, but you should be careful about relying on them for regular use since codeine belongs to the narcotic family (see below). Codeine often causes constipation, which might cause further discomfort, especially if your endometriosis affects your bowel.

If over-the-counter medicines don't help, or give you stomach upsets or constipation, your GP may be able to prescribe a stronger drug or one with fewer side effects.

Prescribed painkillers

If aspirin or ibuprofen don't help endometriosis pains, your GP may offer you a stronger anti-inflammatory drug, e.g. mefenamice acid (Ponstan). Some sufferers have found naproxen (Synflex) helpful. These drugs also have a tendency to irritate the stomach-lining (see advice above).

Your GP may suggest stronger drugs related to codeine such as dihydrocodeine (DF 118) or dextromoramide, although they can also produce constipation and shouldn't be used daily because of the risk of dependence. A similar drug, dextropropoxyphene, is included with paracetamol in Distalgesic.

Equagesic is sometimes prescribed for pain. It includes aspirin and ethoheptazine citrate, another mild pain-reliever, and meprobamate, a tranquilliser that can cause addiction if used regularly. Pentazocine (Fortral and in Fortagesic) may be recommended for moderate to severe pain since its strength lies between that of codeine and morphine. However, it tends to cause nausea and vomiting. It is more effective when injected, but can cause hallucinations, and regular injection has resulted in dependence.

Your doctor will probably be unwilling to prescribe something stronger for any length of time because many moderate and severe painkillers are narcotics, well-known for their tendency to cause physiological addiction (when the body develops a physical need for the drug) and psychological dependence (when people have a craving and feel they can't cope without it) if used regularly. They may also produce tolerance, when an increasing dose is needed to produce the same effect.

If you suffer from severe pain, you may remember the painkilling effects of morphine or pethidine used after surgery and wish your doctor could prescribe something similar.

However, the more effective a drug is for killing pain, the more likely it is to cause side effects or addiction. Morphine and related narcotics are not suitable for regular use because patients can become dependent after two to four weeks, even on low doses, and severe withdrawal symptoms can occur if treatment stops.

Tranquillisers, sleeping pills or anti-depressants can also be prescribed for chronic pain. This does not mean you are mentally ill or that your endometriosis is psychosomatic; emotional states contribute to how we experience pain, so these drugs can help pain temporarily by reducing anxiety or depression, or encouraging sleep. However, long-term use of drugs such as Valium or Mogadon can reduce your pain tolerance, interfere with sleep and cause depression. Some sleeping pills and painkillers combine to produce more rather than less pain if taken together, though long-term use of drugs such as Valium, Ativan and Mogadon can lead to addiction.

PROBLEMS WITH PAINKILLERS

Relying on painkillers can be a very frustrating process of juggling the benefits and side effects of different drugs, and there are no miracles.

If possible I take 10 ml Valium (knocks me out), go to bed and pray I don't wake up. This is obviously only possible at night. During the day I take Distalgesic (not the best, makes me sleepy and 'heavy').

If you are being prescribed a painkiller which you feel isn't helping enough, talk to your doctor. You might gain relief from trying a different type of painkiller (e.g. an anti-inflammatory such as Ponstan or Synflex, or codeine-type drugs such as Distalgesic or DF 118 for the worst days). Equally, if the painkilling effect is good but you have bad side effects, another drug could be more suitable.

If you use prescribed painkillers regularly, you may be alarmed to read about the side effects and dangers mentioned above. If the drug has not caused problems, you are probably one of the majority for whom it is all right. You can get further information from the *British National Formulary*, but talk to your doctor if you are worried. If you are taking a drug regularly which may be addictive, try not taking it for a bit. If symptoms such as pains, cravings, nervousness, etc., develop, start taking the drug again and consult your doctor immediately for advice and support in withdrawing from it slowly. This chapter suggests several alternative ways of controlling pain, so you will not be left stranded.

DLPA: a nutritional painkiller

DLPA is a mixture of two forms (known as *D*- and *L*-) of phenylalanine, an amino-acid constituent of food proteins. It has been found to reduce pain when taken regularly, it is thought, by blocking enzymes which destroy endorphins, the body's own painkillers. Endometriosis sufferers have found DLPA helpful, sometimes for specific components of their pain.

> I can't tell you how glad I am that a friend passed on details of the DLPA treatment. My chronic back pain has not responded to steroid injections, morphine or pethidine drugs. (I am unable to take codeine or aspirin). Already, the general level of pain is lowered and I can now 'pace myself' each day without being overwhelmed by pain. This is the best news in three dreadful years.

Tablets are taken for several weeks, rather than when you are in pain. The initial dose of 375 mg twice daily is gradually increased to 2 × 375 mg three times a day. Once this dose is reached, pain relief should start within a few days and persist for two to three weeks after the end of treatment.

DLPA is non-addictive and you don't have to take longer and larger doses for the same effect. A few sufferers have reported severe indigestion as a side effect. DLPA should not be used in pregnancy, and those with high blood pressure should take it after meals.

DLPA can be used with any existing treatment, including aspirin or anti-inflammatory drugs. Vitamins B6 and C appear to make DLPA more effective if they are taken at the same time. If you can't get DLPA locally, it can be obtained through the Endometriosis Society.

Alternative remedies

Endometriosis sufferers report that various supplements help pain, e.g. selenium, evening primrose oil and calcium (see

Chapter 5). Several home remedies are recommended, but you should consult a medical herbalist or homoeopath for more specific advice.

- A pinch of powdered ginger or a few shreds of root ginger in a cup of boiling water sipped at regular intervals (sweeten with honey if desired) relieves spasms and improves circulation.
- One teaspoon of essence of peppermint, eight teaspoons of oil of orange, eight teaspoons of oil of ginger, in a pint of water. One tablespoon to be taken in a glass of hot water for period pain.
- Thyme tea is also advocated for gynaecological pain.
- Angelica root is a traditional remedy from China, boiled as a kind of soup and taken throughout the cycle.

PHYSICAL TREATMENTS FOR PAIN

Transcutaneous electrical nerve stimulation

Transcutaneous electrical nerve stimulation (TENS) is based on the idea that nerves can be stimulated to prevent pain messages from the damaged site reaching the brain. A small battery-operated device generates a series of pulses which stimulate nerves via two electrodes stuck on the skin with conducting paste. The process is painless and studies have shown that 65–95 per cent of patients with a variety of conditions benefit in the short term, with 30–50 per cent of people still experiencing relief months later. A study of women with pelvic pain, using a similar method for one hour daily for one and a half months, showed 30–50 per cent relief after a week and 60–80 per cent after 20 treatments.

TENS appears to work best for persistent pain. Side effects are minimal – sometimes a slight rash from the electrode paste – although it should not be used if you are pregnant or have a pacemaker (see manufacturer's instructions). The equipment is not easy to get on the NHS (but do ask your GP), so you may have to buy one. TENS machines are about £60 (1988), but it may be worth it compared to endless bottles of aspirin and continuing pain. Some medical equipment suppliers (see Yellow Pages) will allow sale or return, or refund part of the purchase price if it does not work for you. Some hospital pain clinics can lend you one to see if it works.

Acupuncture

The ancient Chinese art of acupuncture is thought to work in a similar way to TENS; it is said to restore energy flows in the body, dispersing pain and allowing healing. Diagnosis before acupuncture treatment is made by feeling pulses in different parts of the body. Treatment then involves stimulating specific points with needles for varying lengths of time. Acupuncture needles are very fine, and skilled insertion is almost painless. The needles may then be rotated or electrically stimulated, or the herb moxa may be burnt over the sites (moxibustion).

In a consumer survey in *Which?* magazine (October 1986), nearly a quarter of 446 people who had used acupuncture for chronic pain said they were cured, almost another half reported improvement and 60 per cent said they would definitely use it again and recommend it to others. Some endometriosis sufferers have found it beneficial: others have not. As with many treatments (including surgery!) you may suffer more before you get better, so don't give up too soon.

For a list of qualified practitioners who will exercise proper safeguards against the spread of disease by needles, write to the Council for Acupuncture (see useful addresses). Doctors who use acupuncture belong to the British Medical Acupuncture Society.

Forms of therapeutic massage

There are several specialist forms of massage, well known for relaxing the body and relieving pain.

Acupressure is a Chinese first-aid technique which uses finger-pressure to stimulate acupuncture points. It was developed into shiatsu by the Japanese. Both have the merit that it is possible to learn to do them yourself, or you can ask a friend to learn. A qualified practitioner will be able to ascertain what pressure points are appropriate for you; for example, try rubbing the point in the hollow just below your knee for period pain – feel around till you find a place that is slightly tender and then rub with the thumb for about 10 minutes.

Reflexology relies on stimulating points on the feet which correspond with the body's organs.

Aromatherapy is a form of massage using essential oils which are believed to have therapeutic properties. Essential oils are sold in many healthfood shops, The Body Shop, etc., but an aromatherapist can give you more specific advice.

Contact community centres, adult education departments, yoga teachers, health farms, gyms and health clubs to find out about local practitioners, courses and workshops.

Heat and cold

Many people find a warm bath, shower, sauna or using a hot-water bottle or heating pad helps pain, and endometriosis sufferers are no exception. And cold is said to be even more effective than heat. Rub a cold object, e.g. a hot-water bottle filled with ice cubes over the painful site. Keep it moving all the time. As soon as your skin feels numb, stop treatment and start moving that part of the body again. It should feel better.

Exercises for pelvic pain

Just as movement is best for a leg cramp, so your pelvic muscles need to be gently exercised rather than being allowed to carry on contracting spasmodically. If possible try the following, rather than curling up in bed.

- Lie on your back with your feet propped up against a wall. Stay there for five to ten minutes.
- Lie on your back on the floor or bed and, keeping one leg still, bring the other one up towards your chin, bending the knee. Hold it there with your hands for a few minutes, then try the other leg.
- Kneel on the floor. Rest your forearms so your elbows are on the floor in front of you, with your head between your arms. Rock gently backwards and forwards with your head alternately between your arms and above your hands.

THE VICIOUS CIRCLE

What do you feel when you are in pain? Do you anticipate more pain? Worry about needing surgery? Remember you have got endometriosis or that you are infertile? Feel angry about your plans being spoilt? Feel guilty about your partner or children having to put up with you? Feel it is unfair and people don't understand what you are going through?

If I am emotionally unhappy, the pain worsens.

At the moment I know that although my chances of pregnancy are small, they would be much better if I could only get rid of the pain for a while. I could then forget my non-pregnant state, relax more and give myself a better chance of conceiving.

The way you feel about your pain can have a considerable effect on its intensity. Pain can be made better or worse by how you respond to it, and yet depression and anxiety are a natural response to being debilitated. You can end up in a vicious circle. This doesn't mean it is your fault if you are in terrible pain or feeling angry or demoralised by it: but it does mean that you can harness the most potent pain-control agent there is – your mind. This may seem unlikely, but it is effective.

What do you do when you are in pain? Do you rub the sore place? Cry? Tell other people and ask them to help? Avoid doing anything that makes it hurt? Get some rest? Take medicine? Go to the doctor? These can be good strategies for short-term pain relief because they give the body a chance to heal itself. But if the pain gets no better or keeps coming back, you need a different approach to prevent you from becoming an invalid, unable to lead a normal life.

Many endometriosis sufferers (and other people who suffer from chronic pain) have found that a change in lifestyle can help to prevent pain occurring, and minimises it when it does. They have learnt to manage their pain by making changes in their daily routine and thinking more positively. Many people find this easier to do if they have support, either from their family, a self-help group or even professional advice from a NHS pain clinic (ask your GP if there is one in your area). The clinic will devise a regime of pain-control techniques and teach you ways out of the vicious circle of feelings and pain. You can try developing your own programme using the following sections.

A PAIN-CONTROL PROGRAMME

Being positive and wholehearted
You can make your life more comfortable and take steps to deal with the pain, but you will have to face the pain and decide to do something positive. This involves accepting that there is no instant cure for your distress, but that you can take many different steps to help yourself.

Most thoughts about pain are negative, which can lead to more anxiety and more pain. If you think you can't cope, you probably won't. But how do you stop understandable feelings of panic?

Research on women due to have gynaecological surgery has shown that a simple exercise where they were asked to list their fears and then revise them more positively helped women feel better about the operation, and they needed fewer painkillers afterwards. So, prior to your next bout of pain, think of things to say to yourself to counteract the inevitable negative feelings. Those based on your previous experience are probably best.

This is killing me.	This isn't going to kill me and if I can get through the next hour, it will ease off a bit.
It is getting worse.	It will get better if I relax.
Painkillers make me feel ill and don't help.	Maybe I can try DLPA or the recommended exercises.

It can be very difficult to give up negative ways of coping if you are confusing your emotional needs with your pain. For example, you may feel people only care about you when you are not well or only ask you how you are feeling when you are in pain. You may only allow yourself to rest when you are in pain, or that may be the only time you ask other people to take over some of your commitments.

Everyone needs to feel cared for whether or not they are in pain. You and your family may have got into the habit of forgetting about your needs unless you are in pain. Try asking your partner or children to get their own meals more often, not just when you are ill. Give yourself a break before the pain gets worse, not when you've collapsed. Ask your partner for love, concern and help when you need it, not just when you are in pain and your partner feels obliged to give it. Do something special together when you're feeling better, so you feel you are giving something in return and not just 'a moaning old ratbag at 27'.

Keeping your mind active
Keep busy. Try to maintain your daily activities as far as possible, especially those you enjoy. It has been found that those who go to bed with period pains are likely to suffer more

than those who try to do things to take their minds off their pain. Reading a book, watching TV, talking to friends are activities more likely to be helpful. At the height of the spasms even singing a song can help distract you from the intensity of the pain.

When the pain is bad, I have to give myself a serious mental talk i.e. if people can fight cancer, why can't I fight this?

This does not mean being stoical and keeping going until you collapse. Endometriosis sufferers need to be kind to themselves by assessing their needs and asking others to help at the right time, instead of just when they are suffering. General support can help you fight the pain when it is bad.

Keeping your body active

Many people cope with chronic pain by becoming increasingly inactive. This can make matters worse since whole groups of muscles can remain virtually unused. Loss of tone in the back and abdominal muscles can then lead to back injuries and strains, causing further painful problems.

I had really awful back pains – usual endometriosis-type pain, but much worse. I was nearly screaming with pain when I tottered into the surgery. It turned out to be lumbago; nothing to do with endometriosis at all.

Exercise prevents these problems, but if you are going to do it regularly, it has to be enjoyable. What about the following? If you find walking, stretching or vibration painful, choose something gentle.

- Aerobics, running and cycling are often recommended for getting you fit and stimulating the flow of endorphins (the body's natural painkillers). Choose this sort of exercise if you don't have too much of a pain-barrier to overcome.
- Walk at your own pace, somewhere you enjoy. Some people recommend getting a dog.
- Yoga is a complete therapy, as well as exercise. Try it if stretching is not too painful. There may be teachers locally.
- Swimming exercises the whole body. The water is supportive, preventing some of the dragging pain you may get when standing or walking. Try the exercises opposite.

Waist swing.
Hold onto the rail. Relax with your legs straight and together. Gently swing your body and legs from the waist down, first to one side, then the other. Keep your upper body and shoulders still. Repeat five times each side and increase to 20.

Waist twist.
Hold onto the rail. Draw your knees up to your chest. Holding this position with your knees pressed together, twist as far as you can to the right. Hold for four or five seconds. Return to middle and then repeat movement to the left. Return to the middle and repeat exercise. Complete sequence five times and increase to 20 times.

Curls-ups.
Hold onto the rail, with arms bent and legs stretched out behind you. Grip your legs together and slowly bend your knees up towards your chest. Hold for four or five seconds. Relax. Repeat exercise. Start with five and increase to 20 times.

- Dancing needn't be at a disco. You can put on your favourite record and be as mild or wild as you like in your own home.
- Alexander technique and Feldenkreiss method are both designed to reduce pain in your daily life by improving posture and muscle tone. There may be classes locally.

Keeping your pelvic-floor muscles in good condition (see Chapter 1) helps avoid some of the painful problems caused by surgery, lack of oestrogen, childbirth and constipation.

Learning to relax

For the first time in my life I feel in control. Now that I have the ability to relax I get so much more out of life and don't spend half my time worrying about what may or may not ever happen.

Relaxation is an invaluable skill for everyone, but it is especially helpful if you suffer from chronic pain. You don't have to find a dark room and half an hour a day where you are uninterrupted, although they will help.

You can learn breathing and muscle tensing and relaxing exercises which you can do anywhere, even stopped at traffic lights in the car, but you will need to spend more time on relaxation if you are going to help chronic pain. You can buy relaxation and pain-control tapes, or there may be relaxation classes locally. Yoga and autogenic training are therapies which teach relaxation.

There are no special clothes or equipment for autogenic training. The therapist guides the group through a set of exercises which warms your limbs, steadies your heartbeat and calms your breathing. After four weeks there was a marvellous lifting of anxiety. I cheered up tremendously. My aches and pains diminished as my muscles unknotted. I was amazed to find that many everyday things which had caused me problems were really quite easy. There have been ups and downs since but perhaps life doesn't get me in the same way. Nothing succeeds like success and if you've had even a week of feeling calm and healthy, you know it can happen again and it will.

This method of relaxation has helped me live with the complaint by reducing pain and releasing additional energy to take up activities to promote my well-being – dancing and painting.

The key to relaxation is breathing. Most of us breathe by inflating the upper parts of our chests. When in distress we breathe more and more shallowly. To relax, you need to take deep, slow breaths, by lowering your diaphragm, rather than raising your ribcage. If you practise this, just taking a few deep breaths will help you to calm down when you feel bad.

Sit comfortably or lie on your back, close your eyes and breathe deeply and slowly. Become aware of each part of your body in turn, beginning with your feet and moving upwards to your head. If a part of your body feels tense consciously relax it. (It helps some people to tense up each group of muscles and then allow them to relax.) Pay special attention to the muscles of your neck, shoulders and face. Now imagine yourself in a pleasant natural setting and concentrate on the details of this special place while continuing to breathe deeply and easily. After some minutes of relaxation, you can gradually let yourself return to your everyday life and open your eyes.

Visualisation

Just as emotional difficulties can promote endometriosis, (see Chapter 8) your mind can also help to make you well. Visualisation seeks to harness your powers of imagination to heal your body. It involves picturing to yourself, in a symbolic way, the processes needed for your life to improve, while you are deeply relaxed. The way you imagine things can be as silly as you like – they only need to have meaning for you and to express as powerfully as possible the goal you are trying to achieve.

Try adding to your relaxation the following exercise to improve your condition: After you have reached a relaxed state and are feeling comfortable, imagine the endometriosis cells in your body. See them weak and confused because they are in the wrong place. Now imagine the purposeful army of white blood cells, your body's natural defenders, flooding in as the blood flow round your pelvis improves. They destroy and dispose of the unwanted cells, tidying up scar tissue and soothing inflammation. Imagine all your organs pink and healthy and your hormones balanced. See yourself healthy and full of energy, getting what you want out of life. After about

10 minutes, gradually allow yourself to return to normal, having assured yourself that you are going to feel better.

Practised regularly at least once a day, this technique can help. It's even helped 'incurable' cancer. But your images should be convincing. If it looks like the endometriosis cells might win or you can't really imagine yourself happy and healthy, you need to consider whether your unconscious mind has reasons for keeping you ill. You can do this best by allowing yourself to fantasise about life without endometriosis as you are relaxing.

You can also use this technique specifically for pain (see box) or for other problems in your life.

VISUALISATION TECHNIQUES FOR PAIN

First relax using your favourite method. Then try one of the following.

- Imagine that your hand is very cold, so that it becomes numb. Now put your hand where the pain is and allow the numbness to soak through your skin to anaesthetise the pain.
- Visualise one of your hands as being your uterus. Concentrate on making the illusion as real as possible. Tense your hand up into a fist and then let the muscles relax, allowing the uterine muscle to relax as well.
- Visualise your pain as an animal. Make it as real as possible. Now have a dialogue with it. Ask it why it is there, what its purpose is and what its message is. Ask what you must do to make it go away. Listen to it and do what it says.

Eating well

Everybody tells you to have a good diet if you want to keep well. Your local clinic or health education department (see under your district health authority in the phone book) will have leaflets on how to reduce fat intake while maintaining adequate protein and vitamin levels.

Pay particular attention to fibre intake – bowel symptoms

are a huge problem with endometriosis sufferers. Fibre can aid constipation and level out fluctuations between diarrhoea and constipation. You don't need bran with everything (too much can make things worse at first), but eat plenty of whole grains, fruit and vegetables.

Try to control your intake of caffeine and alcohol as these can add to your body's physical reactions to stress and may exacerbate pain in the long run.

Enjoying sex again

Endometriosis can make sex hell for you, and not much fun for your partner. This seems to be a particular problem in heterosexual relationships, because penetration can produce sharp pains deep in the pelvis or leave women feeling 'as if I've been kicked' for some time afterwards. Other women find orgasm starts painful contractions, which may be worse during drug treatment if the uterine muscle becomes hypersensitive. Painful sex (dyspareunia) is one of the most difficult problems endometriosis sufferers and their partners have to face, but there are things you can do to help yourselves – and each other.

Painful sex is a shared problem which you need to talk about. You may be the one in pain, but your partner doesn't want to hurt you. You are both likely to feel angry and frustrated by the endometriosis, anxious about making love and worried that the problem will cause you to drift apart. Your expectations of each other may change, without either of you knowing what the other is feeling.

He always used to say 'I love you' during sex. I didn't want him to say it any more (or even make love to me). How could he mean it when he knew it hurt me? When we talked I realised that he hadn't stopped loving me because of the endometriosis, and naturally still had sexual feelings, but hated the idea of hurting me. Together we found it was much better when I was on top; penetration wasn't as deep and I was more in control and able to move if I thought it was going to hurt.

Your partner may feel rejected, or that you don't enjoy sex any more, when the truth is that you don't enjoy the pain, rather than sex itself or being with your partner. You may fear your partner will leave you for a woman without endomet-

145

riosis. You can only get each other's reassurance if you talk about your fears. Talking can also help you work out ways to continue sharing your sexuality.

Give yourselves more time and ask each other for encouragement and stimulation. Working together to make sure you are sexually aroused before penetration can help enormously – you become lubricated, your vagina elongates and the cervix moves higher up so there is less impact on it and other pelvic organs. You are less likely to contract the muscles at the vaginal entrance involuntarily (vaginismus). Vaginismus may develop if you have experienced a lot of pain. It can make penetration uncomfortable or even impossible, but often improves when you begin to feel more relaxed.

Working together to make sure your partner is aroused can help him feel less rejected – he will find it easier to be more caring if he feels you are encouraging his sexuality rather than trying to dampen it down. Remember there is no rush, and penetration isn't everything. It can be fun to delay it as long as possible, or rule out penetration for several weeks while you experiment with other ways of making love. This will help you regain confidence in each other and even rejuvenate your lovemaking. If penetration is still painful later on, then you will feel able to share your sexuality in different ways while you are getting treatment.

Several physical problems, apart from your endometriosis, may be contributing to your pain, and are worth checking. Lack of lubrication when you are sexually aroused may be due to lack of oestrogen because of drug treatment, breastfeeding, removal of your ovaries or the natural menopause. Try KY Jelly from the chemists as a lubricant, or rub a little vitamin E oil into your vagina. Your doctor may prescribe oestrogen creams or hormone replacement therapy if you are menopausal (see page 57). Pain in your vagina or vulva could be due to an infection of thrush, which is common during hormone treatment. Ask your doctor to check in case you need treatment.

You may have the added problem of infertility, and desperately want a baby. Your sex life may become governed by your menstrual cycle and the need for penetration; you can then get into a vicious circle where sex becomes too unhappy and painful. Consider talking to your doctor about artificial insemination (using your partner's sperm) to take the pressure off your sexual relationship while giving you a chance to conceive.

If you feel your relationship will not be helped by any of the above, then you (and your partner) may need outside support to help you sort out the difficulties that painful sex is causing. You may feel it would be too embarrassing to talk to someone else about your problems, but many people have been helped by seeing a counsellor. And counselling may be able to help sort out problems in your relationship which may be contributing to the pain.

Talking to someone can also help you if you are single and previous experiences of painful sex are preventing you from even wanting to start a new relationship. Try asking your GP to refer you, or contact the local branch of Relate (used to be called the Marriage Guidance Council) or Family Planning Association. Both Relate and the FPA are happy to help unmarried or gay women.

Good luck!

RECOMMENDED READING

For detailed information on relevant subjects such as hysterectomy, infertility, the menopause, alternative approaches and pregnancy, try a good bookshop or writing to some of the organisations whose addresses have been listed. The following list emphasises references which specifically cover endometriosis or which you may not readily come across:

M. Ballweg and S. Deutsch, *Overcoming Endometriosis*, Arlington, 1988

M.W. Booker, 'Endometriosis', *British Journal of Hospital Medicine*, May 1988

L.J. Breitkopf and M.G. Bakoulis, *Coping with Endometriosis*, Thorsons, 1988

M.A. Bruhat and M. Canis (eds.) 'Endometriosis', *Contributions to Gynaecology and Obstetrics* Volume 16, Karger Barle, 1987

M.G. Brush and E.M. Goudsmit (eds.), *Functional Disorders of the Menstrual Cycle*, John Wiley and Sons, 1988

British National Formulary published annually by British Medical Association and The Pharmaceutical Society of Great Britain.

P. Connolly, *The Candida Albicans Yeast Free Cookbook*, Fountain Press, 1986

A. Fox and B. Fox *DLPA – An End to Chronic Pain and Depression*, Longshadow, 1985

Judy Graham, *Evening Primrose Oil*, Thorsons, 1984

E. Grist, *A Woman's Guide to Alternative Medicine*, Fontana, 1986

K. Hunt and M. Vessey 'Long-term effects of postmenopausal hormone therapy', *British Journal of Hospital Medicine*, November 1987

S.H. Kennedy, N.D.W. Soper, O.A. Mojiminiyi, B.J. Shepstone and D.H. Barlow, 'Immunoscintigraphy of ovarian endometriosis: a preliminary study', *British Journal of Obstetrics and Gynaecology 95*, 693–697, 1988

'Endometriosis – continuing conundrum', *British Medical Journal 281*, 889–890, 1980

National Consumer Council, *Patients' Rights*, HMSO, 1983

D.T. O'Connor, 'Endometriosis', *Current Reviews in Obstetrics and Gynaecology*, Volume 12, Churchill Livingstone, 1987

J. Older, *Endometriosis*, Scribners, USA, 1984. Only available through the Endometriosis Society.

J. Pleshette, *Cures that Work*, Century Arrow.

J. Rakusen, *The Menopause: A guide for women of all ages*, Health Education Authority, 1987

E. Trimmer, *Selenium*, Thorsons, 1988

L. Wallace and A. Broome (eds.) *Psychology and Gynaecological Problems*, Tavistock, 1984

G.D. Ward 'Endometriosis: an overview' *British Journal of Clinical Practice*, Symposium supplement *24*, 34, 1983

K. Weinstein, *Living with Endometriosis*, Addison-Wesley, USA, 1987. Only available through the Endometriosis Society.

P. Westcott, *Alternative Health Care for Women*, Thorsons, 1987

E.A. Wilson (ed.), *Endometriosis*, Alan R. Liss Inc., USA, 1987

Newsletters, 1–50, of the Endometriosis Society include information on its survey and follow-up of 300 women reporting problems with danazol (Kay Adcocks), 1981–9

USEFUL ADDRESSES

A stamped addressed envelope is welcomed when you make
any enquiry.

Endometriosis Society
65 Holmdene Avenue
Herne Hill
London SE24 9LD
Access to up-to-date information, list of local self-help
groups, regular newsletters, workshops etc.

Health Education Authority Library
Hamilton House
Mabledon Place
London WC1H 9TX
01-631 0930

Chapter 2: Understanding Endometriosis

Community Health Council
Look up your local CHC in the phone book for information
and advice about your rights in the health service.

The Patients Association
11 Dartmouth Street
London SW1H 9BN
Help with your rights, making complaints etc.

Chapter 4: Surgical Treatments

Hysterectomy Support Group
11 Henryson Road
London SE4 1HL
Self-help group meetings, information and newsletter.

National Osteoporosis Society
Barton Meade House
PO Box 10
Radstock
Bath BA3 BYB
(0761) 32472
Leaflets and newsletter.

Association of Chartered Physiotherapists in Obstetrics and
Gynaecology
18 Old North Road
Kempsey
Worcester WR53
Send SAE for leaflet on pelvic exercises.

Women's Health Information Centre
52–54 Featherstone Street
London EC1
01-251 6580
A wide range of information available including more on the
menopause and local self-help groups.

Women's Health Concern
PO Box 1629
London W8 6AU
01-601 6669
Range of publications including booklet on the menopause,
and advice on counselling facilities.

Chapter 5: Alternative Approaches
Some of these organisations make a small charge for their
information.

Community Health Foundation
188 Old Street
London EC1
01-251 4076
Programme of courses and workshops on macrobiotics,
shiatsu etc.

Dr Edward Bach Centre
Mount Vernon
Sotwell
Wallingford
Oxon OX10 0PZ
General information, order form for remedies and booklist.

British Naturopathic and Osteopathic Association
6 Netherall Gardens
London NW3
Information and list of registered practitioners.

Positive Health Centre
101 Harley Street
London W1
01-935 1811
Courses in autogenic training.

National Institute of Medical Herbalists
41 Hatherley Rd
Winchester
Hampshire

Candida albicans Advice Group
P.O. Box 89
East Grinstead
West Sussex RH19 1YY
Specific advice on anti-candida diet, booklist and newsletter.

British Homoeopathic Association
27a Devonshire Street
London W1
Advice about obtaining homoeopathy on the NHS.

The Society of Homoeopaths
2 Artizan Road
Northampton
NN1 4HU
0604 21400
List of homoeopaths who are not doctors (and therefore cannot practise on the NHS). Information on homoeopathy in pregnancy and childbirth.

The Traditional Acupuncture Society
11 Grange Park
Stratford-upon-Avon
Warwickshire CV37 6XH

British Acupuncture Association and Register
34 Alderney Street
London SW1V 4EU

The Council for Acupuncture
Suite 1
19a Cavendish Square
London W1M 9AD
Send £1.50 (1988 prices) for a list of practitioners.

Register of Traditional Chinese Medicine
7A Thorndean Street
London SW18

Shiatsu Society
19 Langside Park
Kilbarchan
· Renfrewshire
PA10 2EP

Council for Complementary & Alternative Medicine
Suite 1
19a Cavendish Square
London W1M 9AD

Institute for Complementary Medicine
21 Portland Place
London W1N 3AF
Provides information on alternative approaches.

Women and Medical Practice
666 High Road
Tottenham
London N17
01-885 2277
Has register of alternative practitioners, information on NHS
and counselling services.

Chapter 6: Endometriosis and Infertility

National Association for the Childless
318 Summer Lane
Birmingham
B19 3RL
021-359 4887
Large organisation offering information and counselling.
Find out about your regional group.

Family Planning Information Service
27-35 Mortimer Street
London W1N 7RJ
01-636 7866
Register of infertility services. Your local office will be in
the phone book.

Parent to Parent Information & Adoption Service (PPIAS)
Lower Boddington
Daventry
Northants
NN11 6YB
0327 60295
A support and information service for families who have or
are planning to adopt.

British Agencies for Adoption and Fostering
11 Southwark Street
London SE1 1RQ
01-407 8800

Parents for Children
222 Camden High Street
London NW1 8QR

Adoption Project
Thomas Coram Foundation
40 Brunswick Square
London WC1 1AZ

National Foster Care Association
Francis House
Francis Street
London SW1
Association of foster parents

Child
'Farthings'
Gaunts Road
Pawlett
Nr. Bridgwater
Somerset
Information and counselling service for members. Main
activity is fund-raising for research.

Chapter 7: Endometriosis and Pregnancy

National Childbirth Trust
Alexandra House
Oldham Terrace
Acton
London W3 6NH

Meet-a-Mum Association
3 Woodside Avenue
London SE25 5DW

Cry-sis
BM Crysis
London WC1N 3XX
Helpline: 01-404 5011
Self-help with crying babies.

The Miscarriage Association
PO Box 24
Ossett
West Yorkshire WF5 9XG
0924 830515

Stillbirth and Neonatal Death Society
28 Falkland Place
London W1M 4DE
01-436 5881

Association for Post-Natal Illness
7 Gowan Avenue
Fulham
London SW6 6RH
01-731 4867

Association for the Improvement in Maternity Services
40 Kingswood Avenue
London NW6

Chapter 8: Understanding Your Feelings

Women's Therapy Centre
6 Manor Gardens
London N7
01-263 6200
Offer therapists, courses and workshops

British Association for Counselling
37A Sheep Street
Rugby CV21 3BX
0788 78328/9
Advice about local counsellors, including those who special-
ise in sexual problems.

RELATE – Marriage Guidance Council
76A New Cavendish Street
London W1
Look up your local branch in the phone book.

Association for Sexual and Marital Therapists
PO Box 62
Sheffield ST3 T6
Can provide a list of therapists.

The Institute of Psychosexual Medicine
11 Chandos Street
London W1
01-580 1043

MIND
22 Harley Street
London W1N 2ED
01-637 0741

Westminster Pastoral Foundation
23 Kensington Square
London W8
01-937 6956
Counsellors who can attend to spiritual needs as well.

Chapter 9: Getting To Grips With Pain

See page 154 for addresses of societies dealing with acupuncture and shiatsu.

Neen Pain Management Systems
Barn Lodge
Gooseberry Hill
Swanton Morley
Dereham
Norfolk NR20 4NR
Can supply a small and easy-to-use TENS machine if you cannot find a local supplier.

INDEX

A Complete Guide to Therapy, 126
activity, 139–42
acupressure, 136–7
acupuncture, 101, 103, 106, 131, 136
adenomyosis (internal
    endometriosis), 12
adhesions, 13, 19, 31, 49, 50, 51, 52,
    62, 69, 86, 89, 90, 129
adoption, 93, 97–8
aerobics, 131
Agnus castus, 61, 75–6
alternative medicine, 77, 134–5
Alternative Medicine Today, 79
alternative medicines, 65–83
American Endometriosis Society, 34
amniocentesis, 104
anatomy, *1, 12*
anatomy, pelvic tilt, *4*
anatomy, retroverted uterus, *4*
anatomy, side view, *2*
angelica root, 135
anger, 114
anti-spasmodic drugs, 131
antibodies, 20
antigens, 20
anxieties, 110
appendectomy, 30
aromatherapy, 136
artificial insemination (AID), 93
aspirin, 130, 131
assertiveness, 26, 115
asthma, 67
autogenic training, 142–3

baby, 105
Belgium, 110, 118

bilateral oophorectomy (removal of
    ovaries), 56, 60
biochemic tissue salts, 73
biopsy, 19
bladder, 2, *2*, 5, 25
bleeding during pregnancy, 102
blood clots, 57
blood tests, 20, 41
body, understanding the, 1–9
The Body Shop, 136
bones, brittle, 56, 61
borage seed oil, 69
bowel, 2, *2*, 5, 12, 13, 25
breastfeeding, 106–7
breasts, 53
Brewer's yeast, 67
British Agencies for Fostering and
    Adopting, 98
British Association for Counselling,
    125
British Medical Acupuncture
    Society, 136
British Medical Journal, 29
buserelin, 45

CA-125 blood tests, 20–21
cabbage, 67
caesarean section, 104
calcitonin, 61
calcium, 71, 61, 134
cancer, 57
Candida albicans, 78–81, 105; diet,
    83; treatments for, 80–81
Candida albicans Advice Group, 80
candidiasis, guide to, 79
'career woman's disease', 30, 115

159

cells, 88
cervical cytology clinic, 28
Chaitow, Leon, 79
Child, 123
Child Guidance Service, 125
childbirth, 104
clinical depression, 117
clinical psychologist, 111
Clomid, 87, 90, 92, 94
co-counselling, 125, 126
coil, 34, 116
colic, 105
Committee on the Safety of
    Medicines, 37
community health council (CHC), 28
A Complete Guide to Therapy, 126
conception, assisted, 91–4
contact lenses, 37
contraception: coil, 34, 116;
    contraceptive pill, 9, 34, 44; inter
    uterine device (IUD), 34
corpus luteum, 8
Council for Acupuncture, 136
counselling, 125
cranial osteopathy, 106
cysts, 13, 49, 57, 62, 86, 90, 121

danazol, 35–41, 54, 68, 72, 105, 121
danazol, side-effects of, 36–8
Danol, 35–41
Decapeptyl, 45
decisions, 119
decisions, guide to making, 120
defaecation, painful, 21
denial of endometriosis, 111–13
Dep-Provera, 43
depression, 16, 54, 57, 95, 115,
    116–17
depression, clinical, 117
depression, postnatal, 105–6
diabetes, 57
diagnosis statements, 29–30
diagnosis tests, 20–21
diagnosis, wrongful, 23
diet, 114–5
DLPA (nutritional painkiller), 134
doctors, referral from, 21–8
dolomite, 37, 71
drugs: effectiveness of, 38–39;
    fertility, 90; in clinical trials, 46–7;

side effects, 36–8, *42*; treatments,
    35–47
Duphaston, 41, 43, 45, 98
dydrogesterone, 45
dysmenorrhoea *see* painful periods
dyspareunia *see* sexual intercourse,
    painful

ectopic pregnancy, 102
eggs, 67
emotions, 24–5, 109–26
endocrine, 119
endometriosis: acceptance of,
    117–18; age of sufferers, *29*;
    and babies, 105; beyond the
    pelvis, 20; causes of, 32–4; chronic
    disease, 41, 109; clinical
    statements, 29–30; common
    disease, 28; cure for, 35; degrees
    of, *18*; denial of, 111–13; destroys
    pelvic anatomy, 86; diagnosis, 16;
    drug treatments, 35–47; fears and
    anxieties, 110–11; helping
    yourself, 119–26; illustration of,
    12; inherited, 30–32; and
    laparoscopy, 17; and lasers, 61–3;
    mild, and infertility, 88; pain,
    127–47; pregnancy, 99–104;
    reaction to, 113; recurrence of, 39;
    religious faith, 123–4; statistics of,
    14, 22, 29; stress, 118–19; support
    of medics, 124–6; symptoms, 13,
    22; theories for, 33;
    understanding, 109–26;
    visualisation to heal, 143–4;
    withdrawal and isolation, 113–14
endometrium, 8, 11, 57
Endometriosis Society, ix, 15, 21,
    38, 40, 55, 80, 85, 96, 119, 123
Endometriosis Society Survey, *22*,
    25, 30, 33, 43, 57, 116
endorphins, 130
episiotomy scars, 104
Eugynon, 30, 44
evening primrose oil, 37, 67–9, 103,
    121, 134
exercises, 61, 130, 137, 140, *141*
exhaustion, 111
eyesight, 37

160

Fallopian tubes, 2, 5, 12, 32, 86, 87
Family Planning Association, 147
family planning clinic, 28
Family Practitioner Committee
  (FPC), 27
fears, 110
Feminax, 131
fertility drugs, 90
fibre, 144–5
fibroids, 28
follicle stimulating hormone (FSH),
  8
Foresight, 100
fostering, 97–8
fungicides, 81

gamete intra-Fallopian transfer
  (GIFT), 85, 91
gammalinolenic acid (GLA), 67
gestrinone, 46–7
ginger, 135
glanolin, 69
gonadotrophin releasing hormone
  (GnRH), 46
goserelin, 45, 46
grief, 111
group therapy, 25, 122
guilt, 115

Hahnemann, Samuel, 76
herbal medicine, 73
herbs, 74–6
homoeopathy, 63, 76–8, 101, 106
hormone imbalance, 33, 109, 119
hormone replacement therapy
  (HRT), 28, 56, 57, 58–9;
  advantages and disadvantages,
  58–9
hormone therapy, 39
hormone treatment, 50, 75, 100
hormones, 5, 8–9, 41
hormones, men, 33
human chorionic gonadotrophin
  (hCG), 9
hysterectomy, 49, 52–5
Hysterectomy Support Group, 55,
  123

ibuprofen, 131
immune systems, disorder in, 119

immunology, x, 33, 86, 88
immunoscintigraphy, 21
implants, 45, 46, 56, 57
in vitro fertilisation (IVF), x, 85, 91
infection, 33
infertility, ix, 13, 16, 21, 26, 38, 75,
  85–98, 123
infertility treatments, 89–94
inflammation, 13, 20, 127
insomnia, 16
inter uterine device (IUD), 34
isolation, 113–14

Ladycare vitamins, 60
laparoscope, 25
laparoscopy, 17–21, 28, 38
laparotomy, 49–51, 89
laser laparoscopy, 61–3
lasers, 49
lethargy, 57
leukotrines, 68
levator ani muscles, (pelvic floor
  muscles), 3, 3
libido (sex drive), 54, 57
linoleic acid, 71
luteinised unruptured follicle
  syndrome (LUFS), 87
luteinising hormone (LH), 8, 44
luteinising hormone releasing
  hormone (LHRH), 44

macrobiotic diet, 78
macrophages (scavenger white blood
  cells), 88
magnesium, 71
Marriage Guidance Council, see
  Relate
massage, 136–7
medical oophorectomy (ovaries), 44
medicines, 131
menopause, 28, 35, 57, 117
menopause, surgical, 60
menstrual cycle, 1, 5–9, 6–7, 13, 19,
  46, 87
menstruation, 28, 36
menstruation, retrograde, 32
metaplasis theory, 32
microsurgery, 51
MIND (Mental Health Association),
  125

minerals, 70–72, 82, 103
miscarriage, 101
misdiagnosis, 23
morning sickness, 103
moxibustion and acupuncture, 136
muscle cramps, 37

nafarelin, 45
narcotics, 130
National Association for the
  Childless, 85, 96, 123
National Health Service (NHS), 125;
  rights of patients, 27
National Health Service Pain Clinic,
  138
National Institute of Medical
  Herbalists, 73, 74
Nature, 76
neurosis, 24

oestrogen, 13, 36, 56, 57
oestrogen creams, 61
oestrogen levels, 8
orgasm, 54, 145
osteoporosis (brittle bones), 56, 61
Osteoporosis Society, 61
ovaries, 1–5, 5, 8, 21, 44, 55–7, 86,
  87, 110, 121
ovulation, 8

pain: ix, 15–16, 21, 40, 53, 66, 68, 70,
  86, 95, 102, 110, 114, 127–47;
  acupuncture, 136; alternative
  medicines, 134; chart, 128; control
  programme, 138–47; control
  techniques, 104; emotions of,
  137–8; exercises for pelvic, 137;
  massage, 136; medicines for,
  131–4; physical treatments for,
  135; relief, 129–31; scale, 26; scale
  chart, 130; visualisation to heal,
  143–4
painful periods, 13
painful sex, 13, 16, 21, 22, 24, 26, 32,
  145
paracetomol, 131
pelvic examinations, 16
pelvic floor muscles, 3, 3
pelvic inflammatory disease (PID),
  19, 25

pelvic organs, 89
pelvic tilt, 4
peppermint, 135
Pergonal, 91
period pains, 21, 23, 24, 53
peritoneum, 3, 11, 13, 51, 86, 127
pethidine, 91
pituitary gland, 5, 8, 67
placebo, 65
postnatal depression, 105–6, 117
pouch of Douglas, 12
pre-conceptual care, 100
pregnancy, 36, 38, 99–104
Premarin, 56, 90
premenstrual syndrome (PMS), 67,
  71, 88, 117
premenstrual tension (PMT), 53, 103
prenatal tissue, 33
Primolut N, 43, 100
progesterone, 8
progestogens, 41, 43–7
prolactin (milk producing hormone),
  106
prostaglandin E1 (PGE1), 67
prostaglandins, 87, 127
Provera, 41, 43, 100
psychological problems, 16
psychosomatic complaints, 24
puberty, 28

reflexology, 136
Relate (Marriage Guidance
  Council), 125, 147
relaxation techniques, 122, 142–3
religious faith, 123–4
resolution, 117
retroverted uterus, 4, 16

safflower oil, 69
salicylate, 131
scar formation, 69
scar tissue, 13, 20, 49
scarring, 127
Schussler system (salt imbalances),
  73
selenium, 70–71, 134
self help groups, 122
sexual intercourse, 145–7
sexual intercourse, painful, 13, 16,
  21, 22, 24, 26, 32

shiatsu, 131, 136–7
singer's voices, 37
skin disorders, 67
smoking, 57
Society of Homoeopaths, 78
sperm transport, 86, 87–8
sterilisation, 30
stress, 24, 118–19
support of medics, 124–6
surgical treatment, 49–63
Sweden, 75
symptoms, 13, *14*, *22*, 25

tampons, 34
thrush, 80
thyme tea, 135
transcutaneous electrical nerve
  stimulation (TENS), 135
twins, 31

United States, ix, 19, 67, 118
urination, 13
uterus, 1–5, 8, 12
uterus, feeling position of, *17*
uterus, retroverted, *4*, 16

Valium, 91
venereal clinic, 28
visualisation, 143–4
vitamin B6, 37, 66
vitamin B complex, 66
vitamin C, 69
vitamin E, 69, 91
vitamin supplements, 72
vitamins, 60, 82, 66–9, 103
vitex agnus castus, 75, 91
voice changes, 37

weight gain, 36
weight loss, 82
Westminster Pastoral Association,
  125
Wheatgerm, 67
Which?, 136
Women's Therapy Centres. 126

yeast, 67, 70, 80
yellow card system, 37

zinc, 72, 91, 104
Zoladex, 45, 46

THE ENDOMETRIOSIS SOCIETY was founded by Ailsa Irving in 1981. It organises self-help groups, participates in and funds research and conducts its own surveys as it aims to raise awareness among women and in the medical profession through publicity and education.